Praise for *A Nurse's Step*
Promoti<

MW00843729

"*A Nurse's Step-By-Step Guide to Academic Promotion & Tenure* will serve as an irreplaceable tool for nurses in tenure track positions nationally and internationally. The book includes clear and helpful step-by-step explanations of common questions and considerations related to tenure and promotion for nurses and others entering higher education in similar fields. I highly recommend this book!"

–Melissa Stormont, PhD
Professor of Special Education
University of Missouri

"This book is well-thought-out and exceptionally detailed, making it a readable and engaging book about the tenure process. The authors skillfully present the numerous aspects of the process and its wide variety within and across institutions. The book stimulates reflection and thinking about personal improvement. The authors succeed in their mission of creating a book that is specifically applicable to nursing while being useful to other academic areas!"

–Rosemary Flanagan, PhD, ABPP
Psychologist/Professor (School Psychology)
Touro College, New York

"The authors have demystified the secrets of tenure by outlining strategic approaches to advancing your academic career. *A Nurse's Step-By-Step Guide to Academic Promotion & Tenure* can provide a road map for creating a reasoned, deliberate path to developing a scholarship and service agenda that addresses tenure guidelines at most academic institutions. With its logical and ordered sequence, this book is the best resource to help navigate the complexities of the tenure process."

–Gwen Sherwood, PhD, RN, FAAN, ANEF
Professor and Associate Dean for Practice and Global Initiatives
University of North Carolina at Chapel Hill, School of Nursing

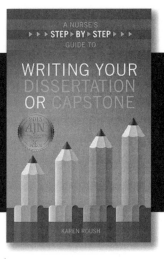
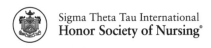
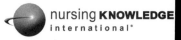

A NURSE'S STEP-BY-STEP GUIDE TO
ACADEMIC PROMOTION & TENURE

CONSTANCE E. MCINTOSH, EdD, MBA, RN
CYNTHIA M. THOMAS, EdD, MS, RNC
DAVID E. MCINTOSH, PhD

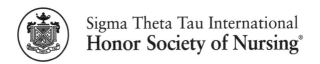

Sigma Theta Tau International
Honor Society of Nursing®

The Honor Society of Nursing, Sigma Theta Tau International (STTI) is a nonprofit organization whose mission is advancing world health and celebrating nursing excellence in scholarship, leadership, and service. Founded in 1922, STTI has more than 135,000 active members in over 90 countries and territories. Members include practicing nurses, instructors, researchers, policymakers, entrepreneurs, and others. STTI's 530 chapters are located at more than 700 institutions of higher education throughout Armenia, Australia, Botswana, Brazil, Canada, Colombia, England, Ghana, Hong Kong, Japan, Jordan, Kenya, Lebanon, Malawi, Mexico, the Netherlands, Pakistan, Philippines, Portugal, Singapore, South Africa, South Korea, Swaziland, Sweden, Taiwan, Tanzania, Thailand, the United States, and Wales. Learn more at www.nursingsociety.org.

Sigma Theta Tau International
550 West North Street
Indianapolis, IN, USA 46202

To order additional books, buy in bulk, or order for corporate use, contact Nursing Knowledge International at 888. NKI.4YOU (888.654.4968/US and Canada) or +1.317.634.8171 (outside US and Canada).

To request a review copy for course adoption, email solutions@nursingknowledge.org or call 888.NKI.4YOU (888.654.4968/US and Canada) or +1.317.634.8171 (outside US and Canada).

To request author information, or for speaker or other media requests, contact Marketing, Honor Society of Nursing, Sigma Theta Tau International at 888.634.7575 (US and Canada) or +1.317.634.8171 (outside US and Canada).

ISBN: 9781940446882
EPUB ISBN: 9781940446899
PDF ISBN: 9781940446905
MOBI ISBN: 9781940446912

Library of Congress Cataloging-in-Publication Data

Names: McIntosh, Constance E., 1967– author. | Thomas, Cynthia M., 1951–
    author. | McIntosh, David E. (David Eugene), 1963– author. | Sigma Theta
    Tau International, issuing body.
Title: A nurse's step-by-step guide to academic promotion and tenure /
    Constance E. McIntosh, Cynthia M. Thomas, David E. McIntosh.
Description: Indianapolis, IN : Sigma Theta Tau International, [2018] |
    Includes bibliographical references.
Identifiers: LCCN 2017036030| ISBN 9781940446882 (print : alk. paper) | ISBN
    9781940446899 (EPUB) | ISBN 9781940446905 (PDF) | ISBN 9781940446912 (MOBI)
Subjects: | MESH: Faculty, Nursing | Universities | Career Mobility |
    Vocational Guidance | Nursing Research | Teaching | United States
Classification: LCC RT71 | NLM WY 19 AA1 | DDC 610.73071/1—dc23 LC record available at
https://lccn.loc.gov/2017036030

First Printing, 2017

Publisher: Dustin Sullivan
Acquisitions Editor: Emily Hatch
Editorial Coordinator: Paula Jeffers
Cover Designer: Rebecca Batchelor
Interior Design/Page Layout: Rebecca Batchelor

Principal Book Editor: Carla Hall
Development Editor: Kezia Endsley
Copy Editor: Charlotte Kughen
Proofreader: Heather Wilcox
Indexer: Larry Sweazy

Dedications

Constance E. McIntosh

This book is dedicated to Dr. David McIntosh, who encouraged me to earn my doctorate. And to Dr. Cynthia Thomas, a dedicated nursing educator who reached out to me when I first started the tenure-track process.

Cynthia M. Thomas

I dedicate this book to Marilyn Ryan and John Thomas, since they were a big part of my journey to earning a doctorate and being tenured.

David E. McIntosh

This book is dedicated to Dr. Betty Gridley, who was my doctoral advisor and dissertation chair. Dr. Gridley took an interest in a young man, saw his potential, and encouraged him to pursue a career in higher education. She is the reason I decided to spend my professional career teaching and conducting research.

Acknowledgments

We extend our deepest gratitude to Dustin Sullivan and Emily Hatch for their support of this book. Consistently, Dustin and Emily showed support for our work through words of encouragement and guidance. We appreciate the STTI Book Approval Committee that believed in this book and believed that its contents would help educators through the process of tenure.

We extend a very heartfelt thanks to our family and friends.

About the Authors

Constance E. McIntosh, EdD, MBA, RN

Connie McIntosh is an Assistant Professor in the School of Nursing at Ball State University. She earned her doctoral degree from Ball State University in special education with a cognate in nursing. McIntosh teaches in the master's degree program. She teaches nursing courses in information technology and management/leadership. Her line of research combines her knowledge of nursing and special education and focuses on the role of school nurses in helping identify, evaluate, and treat children with special needs (e.g., autism spectrum disorder) and the school nurse as an essential leader of the school administrative team. She has published numerous refereed articles and has conducted national presentations. She is currently on a tenure track. McIntosh has been a member of Sigma Theta Tau International for 10 years and has served in various chapter leadership roles. She recently coauthored a book titled *A Nurse's Step-by-Step Guide to Transitioning to the Professional Nurse Role*, published by the Honor Society of Nursing, Sigma Theta Tau International (STTI).

Cynthia M. Thomas, EdD, MS, RNC

Cynthia Thomas is an Associate Professor in the School of Nursing at Ball State University. She earned a doctoral degree from Ball State University in the School of Adult, Higher, and Continuing Education. Thomas teaches management/leadership in three nursing programs: undergraduate, RN to BSN, and the master's degree program. Her primary research focus is the transition from student to the professional nurse role and simulation development and implementation. Thomas, in conjunction with coauthors, recently published *A Nurse's Step-by-Step Guide to Transitioning to the Professional Nurse Role* through STTI. She has had 23 peer-reviewed publications and 38 presentations at national and international nursing conferences. She has served as President of STTI's Beta

Rho Chapter for the past 4 years and the Educational Practices Team Chair for the NLN/Jeffries Simulation Framework Project, and she has served on many other committees at the local and international levels.

David E. McIntosh, PhD

David McIntosh is a full Professor and the David and Joanna Meeks Distinguished Professor of Special Education at Ball State. He received his undergraduate degree from Hanover College (1986). He received a master of arts degree (1987), an educational specialist degree (1987), and the doctor of philosophy (1990) from Ball State. He currently serves as the Executive Director of the Center for Autism Spectrum Disorder. McIntosh also is the Director of the Autism Summer Day Camp. He is the Editor-in-Chief of *Psychology in the Schools*, an interdisciplinary journal that publishes manuscripts focusing on issues confronting schools and children. McIntosh is Board Certified by the American Board of Professional Psychology, a Fellow of the American Psychological Association—Division 16, and a Fellow of the American Academy of School Psychology. He has served as President for the American Academy of School Psychology and as President of the American Board of School Psychology. McIntosh is a recipient of the Benny Award for service to Ball State University. He publishes extensively in the area of psychological and educational assessment of children and adolescents with learning, emotional, and disruptive behavior disorders. He also publishes in the area of identification and treatment of autism spectrum disorder. McIntosh has published more than 70 refereed articles and book chapters. He has received more than $2 million in external funding over the course of his career to support research, students, and academic programs.

Table of Contents

Introduction

Many faculty enter higher education with limited knowledge of the promotion and tenure process. In fact, new faculty often spend little time thinking about promotion and tenure during the application, interview, and hiring processes. If faculty do ask questions related to promotion and tenure during the interview, they tend to be fairly general—for example, "What are the expectations for promotion and tenure?" "How long does it typically take for a faculty member to be promoted or tenured?" "Do faculty receive a raise when being promoted?" These are all common questions. In response, answers tend to be general and noncommittal, leaving the prospective faculty member confused or hesitant to press for clarity. Instead, prospective faculty tend to focus on more comfortable topics, such as negotiating salary, identifying potential courses they might teach, determining service and research expectations, and understanding the nursing curriculum.

This book was developed to assist not only beginning faculty but faculty at all stages of the promotion and tenure process. The authors, Constance McIntosh, Cynthia Thomas, and David McIntosh, represent more than 50 years of experience in higher education. Because this book provides information and guides for beginning professors as well as professors seeking promotion to full professor, it was important for the book's authors to represent different stages of the promotion and tenure process. Specifically, Constance McIntosh, Assistant Professor, is currently earning tenure, just completing her fourth-year review; Cynthia Thomas, Associate Professor, earned tenure a few years back and is working toward promotion to full professor; and David McIntosh is a distinguished Professor with more than 27 years in higher education.

In developing this book, it become clear that, although there was a significant amount of research and articles published related to the history of tenure, the need for tenure, the scholarship of tenure, legal challenges to promotion and tenure, and the continually changing landscape of promotion and tenure, there was minimal information available on how to assist faculty who are pursuing promotion and tenure. Therefore, the book's primary focus is to provide a practical guide for understanding and navigating the promotion and tenure process without understating that promotion and tenure is a complex, often stressful, process. The authors' goal is to take some of the mystery and anxiety out of promotion and tenure. By helping readers gain a better understanding of how to become more educated about promotion and tenure, how to ask the right questions, and how to balance teaching, research, and service, readers can become more confident as they move through the promotion and tenure process. The book also provides suggestions on how to improve instruction, research, and service for faculty who are struggling with promotion and tenure. Throughout the book are bullet points and sidebars to stress important points. Checklists are included to assist readers during the interview and yearly promotion and tenure-review process. Several checklists on teaching, research, and service also have been developed to assist readers in identifying strategies and developing a plan for meeting the promotion and tenure requirements at their universities.

Although nursing faculty will find the book useful as they progress through the promotion and tenure process, faculty representing other disciplines (e.g., education, psychology, economics, and so on) should also find this book helpful. Therefore, encourage your colleagues and other educational professionals to read this book. Because turnover is very expensive, higher education wants its tenure-track employees to be successful, but institutions do not always have the resources to "hand-hold" their faculty. Encourage your college or university to purchase this straightforward solution for every tenure-seeking faculty member.

There is a strong reason to believe this book will increase your understanding of the different aspects of tenure and provide you with helpful checklists on "what to do" and "what not to do." However, there is no guarantee that these methods will earn you tenure in your own institution. The very best to you as you move through your own tenure process. Thank you, again, for purchasing and reading this book.

Note that by the nature of this material, all the lists included in this book are examples and do not claim to be conclusive or complete.

WHAT IS THE PURPOSE OF TENURE?

ELEMENTS OF TENURE

1. Ensures academic freedom

2. Provides protection from external pressures

3. Offers protection from internal pressures

4. Ensures an environment of creative stability

5. Serves the long-term interests of universities and society

What Is Tenure?

Tenure is a practice defined by a set of protocols that have been created and enhanced over time. They are intended to ensure professional academics' continued involvement in defining the academic mission of colleges and universities as well as to ensure that colleges and universities observe procedural due process in making faculty appointments ("tenure-track" appointments) that may lead to continuous appointment. This includes promoting or dismissing faculty who are eligible for continuous appointments and dismissing faculty who have been awarded continuous appointments (Teichgraeber, 2014).

Some institutions recognize tenure and promotion in rank based on expertise in one of four areas and/or contributions in others: research, teaching, service, and practice. Although other universities expect excellence in all three areas of research, teaching, and service, some institutions also provide opportunities for advancement in rank in non-tenure positions. It is essential that you explore all the possibilities at the institution where you are seeking a tenured position.

Tenure continues today to be a very competitive process, as hundreds of PhD/EdD graduates are seeking a single position in some departments on college and university campuses, and tenure is granted based on judgments about the contributions the faculty make during the tenure probationary period (Groves, 2013). Also, the tenure requirements, while often vague, are being increasingly made more rigorous (Groves, 2013).

Ehrenberg and Zhang (2005) believe that tenured faculty aid in and preserve the intellectual paradigm of academia and make for a better experience for students. Research has indicated that non-tenured faculty negatively affect the five- to six-year graduation rate of students and may result in declining admissions and grade inflation. Tenured faculty tend to be more concerned about academic excellence than business profits (Cameron, 2010; Ehrenberg & Zhang, 2005).

As Curtis and Jacobe (2006, p. 16) state, "A lack of tenured faculty would be detrimental to the higher education standards in America." Although there are some, such as Finkelstein and Schuster (2001), who believe that tenure promotes lethargy, others, such as Walden (1980), find that tenured faculty are quite prolific in scholarly productivity after tenure is granted. Tenured faculty also serve as mentors and role models to younger faculty, safeguarding academic freedom and ensuring that students receive a quality education (Cameron, 2010).

THE BOYER MODEL

Many universities follow the Boyer Model when establishing policies and guidelines related to promotion and tenure. The Boyer Model is an academic model with four categories: 1) scholarship of discovery, which includes original research; 2) scholarship of integration that involves interprofessional/interdisciplinary collaboration; 3) scholarship of application (i.e., service); and 4) scholarship of teaching and learning. For a complete discussion and overview of the Boyer Model, go to https://depts.washington.edu/gs630/Spring/Boyer.pdf.

This website leads the reader directly to the PDF of Ernest L. Boyer (1990) titled "A Special Report: Scholarship Reconsidered Priorities of the Professoriate," published by the Carnegie Foundation: For the Advancement of Teaching.

Our readers might want to do a literature review—there are several articles on the Boyer Model—and numerous institutions outline their perspectives and philosophy of the Boyer Model online.

The History of Tenure

If tenure is what you are seeking, it is important to understand the history, including the original reasons why tenure was developed and the overall purpose of tenure. A historical perspective is helpful when making a decision about whether tenure is the professional path that you want to take. Americans, particularly outside academia, may misunderstand the reasons for tenure in U.S. educational institutions.

Not all faculty hold tenure, and tenure does not give faculty the right to not do their jobs. Currently about 30 percent of faculty at U.S. institutions of higher education hold tenure or are qualified to earn tenure. The remaining faculty are considered full-time or part-time in nontenure positions (Hibel & Scholtz, 2016). Essentially, tenure was established to secure the "academic freedom" of faculty to conduct research and teach without restraints from universities and the general public (Mangrum, 2014). Tenure was also established to ensure a contractual relationship between the tenured faculty and the university or college that was enforceable by a court of law (Byse & Joughin, 1959).

Although many individuals within and outside the university setting perceive tenure as a lifetime appointment, there is a general lack of understanding as to why tenure is essential to universities, society, and education in general. Critics of tenure often cite that tenure ultimately leads to lower productivity in the areas of research and teaching. However, several studies have been published that demonstrate that most tenured faculty continue to maintain high levels of scholarly productivity and continue to make significant contributions throughout their careers (Allen, 1996, 2000; Bonzi, 1992; Harrison, 2006; Nikolioudakis, Tsikliras, Somarakis, & Stergiou, 2015). Unfortunately, the public and legislators make broad statements and generalizations regarding the productivity of tenured faculty with little or no support for their statements. The impression is that tenured faculty are quietly sitting at home (or at their beach houses), enjoying a big salary with little to no interaction with students. This view cannot be further from the truth. Although a very small percentage (less than 1%) of faculty might demonstrate decreases in productivity, the majority continue to be quite productive and are highly engaged in instruction.

In fact, most faculty choose higher education as a career because they are highly committed to teaching, research, and professional service activities. Faculty choose career paths in higher education not for the salaries (which tend to be significantly lower compared to their colleagues within the private sector) but for the intellectual stimulation and the opportunity to make advances in their chosen disciplines.

The Importance of Tenure

As mentioned, tenure originated to ensure academic freedom and to protect scholars from external (e.g., legislators, funding agencies, religious organizations, etc.) and internal (e.g., powerful administrators, other tenured faculty, private donors, etc.) pressures.

Tenure allows faculty to have academic freedom when teaching and conducting research that can lead to advancements in pedagogy, technology, and medicine, or changes in political views, employment, and industry. Although the preceding list is not exhaustive, it demonstrates the importance of an academic environment that allows faculty to question and study current perspectives without fear of reprisal or pressure to conform to current thinking. Just think—where would the world be today if Albert Einstein had not had the freedom to discover relativity or sociologists had not conducted the Middletown studies?

Without tenure, it would be more difficult for faculty to express opinions to ensure students are exposed to different perspectives while teaching or to conduct specific lines of research without fear of reprisal or losing their jobs.

WHAT IS ACADEMIC FREEDOM?

According to the American Association of University Professors (AAUP, n.d.), *Academic Freedom* has three main distinct parts to it:

- "Teachers are entitled to full freedom in research and the publication of the results, subject to the adequate performance of their other academic duties; but research for pecuniary return should be based upon an understanding with the authorities of the institution.

- "Teachers are entitled to freedom in the classroom in discussing their subject, but they should be careful not to introduce into their teaching a controversial matter that has no relation to their subject. Limitations of academic freedom because of religious or other aims of the institution should be clearly stated in writing at the time of the appointment.

- "College and university teachers are citizens, members of a learned profession, and officers of an educational institution. When they speak or write as citizens, they should be free from institutional censorship or discipline, but their special position in the community imposes special obligations. As scholars and educational officers, they should remember that the public might judge their profession and their institution by their utterances. Hence they should at all times be accurate, should exercise appropriate restraint, should show respect for the opinions of others, and should make every effort to indicate that they are not speaking for the institution" (p. 2).

Tenure provides a much-needed cultural stability! Without tenure, universities would find it difficult to attract and retain faculty. Tenure encourages faculty to stay at a specific institution, complete research, and mentor the next generation of faculty. Many universities were established with specific missions (e.g., engineering, medicine, teaching, music, etc.), and attracting and retaining the best faculty is crucial to ensuring continued advancements that will have an impact on society.

Tenure Does Not Mean Employment for Life

Although tenure provides certain protections and helps ensure academic freedom, it does not necessarily translate to a guaranteed job for life. As noted, it is a common misconception among the public, and even faculty, that tenure is granted for life. It is astounding how many faculty state, "Administration cannot do anything to me; I am tenured." Besides sounding quite arrogant, the statement cannot be further from the truth.

Faculty are encouraged to closely read the university handbook and human resource policies.

 It is a common misconception that tenure guarantees a job for life.

Most policies address faculty misconduct, ethical violations, chronic low productivity, and university response to any outside illegal activities. It would be hard to imagine tenured faculty members maintaining university employment if they did not show up for classes during most of the semester, were caught plagiarizing several major research studies, or were discovered to be selling illegal drugs to students on campus. Universities typically have policies and procedures in place to terminate a tenured faculty member, if needed.

Although rare, universities can release faculty due to a financial crisis or financial exigency. *Financial exigency* refers to "a financial crisis that fundamentally compromises the academic integrity of the institution as a whole and that cannot be alleviated by less drastic means than the termination of tenured faculty appointments" (American Association of University Professors, 2014, p. 1). Again, the termination of tenured faculty is extremely rare; however, when it does occur, the university typically establishes a protocol for terminations. For example, a university may target faculty in programs with small numbers of students, provide incentives for early retirements, or base termination on seniority.

Post-Tenure Review

Many institutions have developed post-tenure review processes focused on ensuring accountability related to teaching, research, and service. The development of post-tenure review often is in response to external pressures (e.g., legislators), which are often in response to public pressure. Unfortunately, it is increasingly more common for state legislators to make state funding contingent on universities' developing and implementing a post-tenure review process. The rigor of the post-tenure review process varies greatly from one institution to another. At some institutions, the post-tenure review process can be as grueling and demanding as the pre-tenure review process, while at other institutions, tenured faculty may only need to demonstrate a minimal level of productivity over a certain period (e.g., publishing one article within a two-year period or consistently demonstrating high course ratings). It is not uncommon for universities to include the following as part of the post-tenure review process:

- A sustained record of publications in refereed journals

- Presentations at national conferences

- External funding or at least attempts to pursue external funding to support research

- Consistently high course evaluations

- Demonstration of continued service at the department, college, and university levels

- National service (e.g., committee member for a national association, editorial board member for a major journal, grant reviewer, etc.)

At some institutions, faculty are reviewed on a yearly basis, while at other institutions, faculty may be reviewed every three or five years.

When faculty are required to submit materials (e.g., publications, course evaluations, service activities, etc.) annually, post-tenure review often is aligned with merit. Consequently, low levels of scholarly productivity, low course evaluations, or minimal service result in small raises. For faculty who are reviewed every three or five years, the process may require them to submit detailed materials with narratives outlining their achievements since the last post-tenure review.

Regardless, the increased focus on post-tenure review appears to be in direct response to public views that there is significant dead weight within higher education, which has been shown *not* to be true. Essentially, post-tenure review is meant to identify the less than 1% of tenured faculty who are considered nonproductive. In addition, most universities have developed remediation and internal resources to assist nonproductive faculty in becoming more engaged in research, teaching, and service. Only after remediation and internal resources have been provided without proven success would institutions tend to move toward termination of tenured faculty.

Pre-Tenure Probationary Period

The majority of institutions require faculty to complete a probationary period prior to being granted tenure. The probationary period is typically between five and seven years but can range from three to nine years. (The latter is rare.) Depending on the institution, the primary focus of the probationary period is to allow tenure-track faculty opportunities to develop and demonstrate excellence in teaching, demonstrate research productivity (e.g., publications, presentations, grant writing, etc.), or both. Although professional service (e.g., membership on department, college, and university committees; journal editorial advisory board memberships; member on professional committees, etc.) also tends to be emphasized during the probationary period, the majority of institutions are more focused on teaching and publications. Most institutions focus on the following during the probationary period:

- Number and quality of publications
- Number and quality of presentations at national conferences
- Quality of teaching
- Service at the department, college, and university levels
- Service at the national level

The idea is that faculty who demonstrate excellence in teaching, research, and service during the probationary period will continue to demonstrate excellence in all three areas once granted tenure and probation. Recall that research (Allen, 1996, 2000; Bonzi, 1992; Harrison, 2006; Nikolioudakis et al., 2015) has shown that for most disciplines, the majority of faculty granted tenure continue to demonstrate high levels of scholarly productivity and service as well as remain excellent instructors.

Stopping the Tenure Clock

The majority of colleges and universities have policies related to stopping the tenure clock. *Stopping the tenure clock* most often refers to when a faculty member requests that a year not count as a tenure-creditable year. When faculty are permitted to request that a year not count as a tenure-creditable year, the university typically has specific procedures and policies that must be followed related to the request. In addition, a university usually articulates specific conditions for which faculty can request that a year not count as a tenure-creditable year. Situations that result in faculty's requesting that a year not count could include:

- A personal illness that results in a leave of absence from the university

- A family member with a chronic illness

- The need to take care of a family member (e.g., taking care of an elderly parent)

- Death of spouse or child

- Another major life stressor

The conditions or situations that faculty are allowed to base a request that a year not count as a tenure-creditable year vary from one university to the next. Also, some institutions allow faculty to request that more than one year not count as a tenure-creditable year. It is important to consider the following:

- Some institutions will only allow faculty to request that one year not count as a tenure-creditable year during the probationary period.

- Other institutions will allow faculty to request that more than one year not count as tenure-creditable years during the probationary period but limit the number of years (typically two or three) a faculty member can request.

- Still others might not limit the number of years faculty can request to not count as tenure-creditable years.

- Some institutions may require faculty to request a Family and Medical Leave Act (FMLA) leave, which essentially stops the tenure clock.

When a request to not count a year as a tenure-creditable year is granted, the faculty member typically is given an additional year toward earning tenure and promotion. Also, the faculty member is typically not required to submit promotion and tenure materials and is not reviewed by the promotion and tenure committee for the year the request is granted. For example, if a faculty member requests that her fifth tenure-creditable year not count due to having an extended chronic illness for most of her fifth year and it is granted, then she would not submit promotion and tenure materials for review, and she would not be reviewed by the promotion and tenure committee. Her fifth-year promotion and tenure review will actually occur during her sixth year at the university. Essentially, her fifth and sixth years will be rolled together as her fifth-year review. Here are a few final thoughts for faculty considering requesting that a year not count as a tenure-creditable year:

- Faculty often believe that they can *only* request that a year not count as a tenure-creditable year if they were not able to perform all aspects of their positions. This is typically not true. For example, faculty who have continued to work (e.g., teach, attend committee meetings) but have not been able to sustain their research due to taking care of a sick family member should consider requesting that the year not count as a tenure-creditable year. Not all areas (i.e., teaching, research, and service) have to be affected when considering a request to stop the clock.

- Mental health issues (e.g., anxiety disorder, major depressive episode, posttraumatic stress disorder, etc.) can influence faculty performance just as much as medical issues. Therefore, faculty should not be hesitant to request that a year not count as a tenure-creditable year if they have had a mental health issue or had to assist family members with mental health issues.

- At times, faculty are hesitant to request that a year not count as a tenure-creditable year. Faculty often worry about what their colleagues will think, consider the request as a failure, or worry that it will influence a later promotion and tenure decision. It is important to note that the majority of universities have developed policies and procedures related to stopping the tenure clock to protect and retain faculty. Therefore, the option to request that a year not count as a tenure-creditable year should be seen as a benefit, just like the health and life insurance benefits offered through the university. Lastly, faculty may be surprised about the number of faculty who request that a year not count as a tenure-creditable year. Essentially, faculty are granted this request more often than we think!

Promotion to Associate

At many institutions, promotion and tenure are aligned. In other words, when faculty apply for tenure, they also are requesting promotion from assistant to associate professor. However, there are some institutions that continue to grant tenure without promotion. Granting tenure without promotion is becoming less common, because institutions take the perspective that if people are tenurable then they also should be promotable. Institutions want to avoid the negative stigma of having tenured assistant professors. Specifically, universities with a Carnegie Doctoral classification are more likely to align tenure with promotion compared to universities with Carnegie Master's, Baccalaureate, and Associate's classifications (see http://carnegieclassifications.iu.edu for an overview and list of Carnegie classified institutions), where it is more likely for assistant professors to be granted tenure without promotion. For many Master's, Baccalaureate, and Associate institutions, the focus is on granting tenure with the goal of retaining highly qualified instructors. Specifically, the focus is on retaining faculty who demonstrate high levels of service and who are exemplary teachers.

When a faculty member is granted tenure and promotion at the associate level, the college or university is making an investment in that individual. The faculty member also is making a commitment to the institution by accepting tenure and the appointment to the associate level. There is an informal agreement that the institution will continue to support and provide the needed resources for the faculty member to be successful in teaching, research, and service, and the faculty member informally agrees to demonstrate scholarly productivity, excellence in teaching, and excellence in service.

At major research institutions, faculty are expected to continue to refine their research with the goal of developing nationally recognized lines of research. Faculty are also expected to begin to pursue external funding to support their research, students, and the university. Associate professors are expected to continue to demonstrate a level of continuous scholarly productivity that ultimately will position them to apply for full professor.

Promotion From Associate to Full Professor

A smaller percentage of faculty pursues the rank of full professor after being promoted to associate compared to the percentage of assistant professors promoted to associate professor. The smaller number of full professors at colleges and universities compared to the number of associate and assistant professors is due to a variety of reasons. The majority of assistant professors must pursue tenure and promotion to associate to retain their positions, which tends to be a significant motivator. Some associate professors will make career changes within higher education, pursuing director, chair, or administrative positions.

At some colleges and universities, there are requirements that associate professors must obtain significant external funding prior to applying for full professor. Many institutions require a clear line of research, as demonstrated by publications, presentations, and grants focused on the same area, prior to supporting a faculty member's application for full professor. Although meeting criteria for promotion to full professor can be daunting, some associate professors never gain the confidence to apply for promotion to full professor, even if they demonstrate high levels of scholarship. Others may fear being evaluated by their peers or fear being turned down for promotion to full.

Interestingly, the majority of universities allow faculty to apply for full professor without risk of termination. Although some institutions allow faculty to apply for full professor each year, it is not uncommon for faculty to be limited in the number of times they can pursue full professor with a given time period (e.g., once every two years, once every five years) at other institutions.

The Tenure Process

Faculty who have earned a terminal degree (PhD, EdD, and in some situations a master's degree) in an academic field of study may be eligible for a tenure-track position. Although we cannot give specific requirements for every higher institution in the United States, we can provide basic generalities that exist among U.S. colleges and universities. There are a limited number of tenure-track positions within an academic department, so in some institutions, competition can be rigorous. Most universities give the title of assistant professor to tenure-track faculty during the probationary period.

The probationary period is a time when the tenure-track faculty demonstrate the ability to participate in scholarly productivity and excellence in teaching. Scholarly productivity (i.e., scholarly activity) encompasses a variety of work, including:

- Original research

- Publishing in peer-reviewed publications

- Presenting work at national and international conferences

- Obtaining grants

These activities are in addition to teaching and service expectations. The expectation is that the faculty will increase productivity in the required areas and demonstrate excellence by becoming an expert in the chosen field (Cameron, 2010; Groves, 2013; Oregon State University, 2014; Siliciano, 2012; University of California Berkeley, 2016).

According to the National Education Association (NEA, 2015), earning tenure comes with the benefit of a right to due process. In other words, after a faculty member is tenured, the university needs to prove incompetence, unprofessionalism, or lack of productivity for a faculty member to lose his or her job. Another reason for faculty being dismissed may include a specific program's or department's being discontinued due to financial reasons for the university. It is challenging to become tenured and for obvious reasons difficult to be terminated once tenured. If tenure is denied, then the faculty member is given an established period of time to move on, but in most universities, faculty may not retain employment. Any time during the probationary period, the university may terminate the faculty, or the faculty may choose to terminate the probationary process without cause.

According to the NEA (2015), one in five tenure-track faculty is denied tenure and thus loses employment each year. A title of associate professor is often bestowed after tenure is granted. Once tenured, faculty are held accountable for continual achievement in areas of scholarly productivity, and work is reviewed in a merit process or post-tenure review.

The *tenure review committee* may be titled differently, depending on the organization, and in many universities, this committee is often referred to as the *promotion and tenure committee*. The committee comprises tenured faculty from within the tenure candidate's department or a combination from within and outside the department. The committee of tenured faculty review the tenure-track faculty's documents of accomplishments over established periodic time frames, make suggestions for improvement, and/or provide documentation of a successful or unsuccessful tenure year during the probationary period. The committee chair and or members should meet with the tenure-track faculty to review progress. The committee should serve to ensure the tenure-track faculty is staying on track and doing quality work. If the tenure-track faculty receives an unsatisfactory tenure year, then an appeal for additional review or decision reversal may be submitted.

Often, year 6 is the time many institutions determine whether the candidate has demonstrated successful progress toward tenure, and the committee formalizes the process with a letter of recommendation to the college dean or university provost, who will then recommend to the institution's board of trustees that tenure be conferred. Many institutions require the candidate to complete the seventh year prior to the granting of tenure. There are also institutions that require independently tenured faculty reviewers from outside the institution as part of the tenure review process and before a final tenure decision is determined.

The process is arduous but can be enriching and rewarding to the faculty. It is important to keep in mind the long-term goal of tenure and not focus so much on the work to obtain tenure. Although the tenure process may slightly differ depending on the institution, it still remains a challenging process that requires much dedication and work to achieve. However, it can be worth the effort!

Issues to Consider Prior to Going on Tenure Line

Some institutions offer non-tenure-line positions (e.g., clinical tracks or contract faculty) that have one-, three-, or five-year appointments. For those individuals who do not want to commit to a tenure-track position, you may want to explore this option. However, for individuals who are interested in a tenure-line position, there are several things to consider.

Professional commitments are equally important when establishing professional connections and when becoming an active member of a professional organization. That being said, these obligations can take more than a fair amount of your time. These professional commitments, although certainly worthwhile, can also play tug-of-war on an already busy work schedule and may prevent work on lines of research. For example, if one of your professional commitments is volunteering as an accreditation-site visitor, you can spend hours, if not weeks, preparing (e.g., reviewing documents) for the site visit. In another example, for those of you whose professional commitments involve serving on the executive board of a national organization as the president, vice president, treasurer, etc. , these can be equally time-consuming. Often, serving on an executive board or committee for a national organization will require travel to annual meetings or conferences. These are the type of commitments that, without a doubt, are beneficial to grow within your profession. However, we must point out how much time, energy, and work are required for such professional endeavors.

Doctoral programs are and should be rigorous in nature, but the most challenging aspect of the process for many students is the dissertation. When doctoral candidates have completed all course work with the exception of their dissertations, they are often referred to as being "all but dissertation" (ABD). The dissertation is the culmination of a research project, including the research completed, the results written, and then eventual submission to the doctoral candidate's committee for review. Then, before the degree is awarded, the doctoral candidate defends the research (i.e., doctoral defense). For many doctoral students, this is a very exciting and rewarding experience, yet for others, the whole process is so daunting and overwhelming that it is not completed.

Farkas (2016) reports that each year, 50% of doctoral students drop out of their programs without completing the work. She explains that there are seven reasons why students drop out of doctoral programs:

- Time-management issues

- Conflicts with others

- Undeveloped thesis

- Burnout

- Issues with writing

- Loss of interest in research

- Feelings of isolation

Dunn (2014) also provides similar reasons doctoral students failed to complete their degrees after interviewing several students who had dropped out of their programs. In addition to the seven common reasons from Farkas (2016), Dunn (2014) hears from former students that financial and family issues as well as a decreased passion for the area of study left them questioning reasons to continue.

Although many students fail to complete their doctoral degrees, there are many others who do complete the degrees and move on to academic positions. If you have not yet completed your doctoral degrees be very cautious about accepting a tenure-line position in academia prior to completing your dissertation.

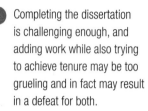 Completing the dissertation is challenging enough, and adding work while also trying to achieve tenure may be too grueling and in fact may result in a defeat for both.

Most likely, these same principles that Farkas (2016) and Dunn (2014) relate may be applied to earning tenure. As we discuss further in this book, there are strategies to employ that will help you be successful, but you are the one who has to do the work. You must set aside time to do the work if you are going to be successful. Conflicts will arise; learn from these experiences and move on. You must have a well-developed thesis to conduct good research.

If you are struggling to write or publish, there are always colleagues and available institutional resources (e.g., writing groups, statistics consultants, writing labs, etc.) willing to assist you with your research, so take advantage of these opportunities. Don't fully isolate yourself from others; people generally want to be helpful and see you be successful. You might also need to collaborate with others to conduct your research, so be open to this concept.

Chapter Checkup

- ❑ Do I have an appreciation and understanding of the purpose and benefits of tenure?

- ❑ Do I understand the specific tenure process at my institution?

- ❑ Am I prepared to build my case for tenure?

- ❑ Does my pre-tenure work accurately reflect my talents and efforts?

- ❑ Do I understand the post-tenure review process at my institution, if there is one?

- ❑ Do I understand the policies and procedures related to requesting that a year not count as a tenure-creditable year?

- ❑ Am I familiar with university resources that can help improve my writing?

- ❑ Am I open to collaborating with other researchers on campus?

- ❑ If my institution allows tenure to be earned in one of four areas (i.e., research, teaching, service, or practice), what will my area of expertise be?

References

Allen, H. L. (1996). Faculty workload and productivity in the 1990s: Preliminary findings. In *NEA 1996 Almanac of Higher Education* (21–23). Washington, DC: National Education Association.

Allen, H. L. (2000). Tenure: Why faculty, and the nation, needs it. *The NEA Higher Education Journal, 16*, 95–110.

American Association of University Professors (AAUP). (2014). Recommended institutional regulations on academic freedom and tenure. Retrieved from https://www.aaup.org/file/RIR%202014.pdf

American Association of University Professors (AAUP). (n.d.). 1940 Statement of principles on academic freedom and tenure. Retrieved from http://www.aaup.org/report/1940-statement-principles-academic-freedom-and-tenure

Bonzi, S. (1992). Trends in research productivity among senior faculty. *Information Processing and Management, 28*(1), 111–120.

Byse, C., & Joughin, L. (1959). *Tenure in American higher education: Plans, practices and the law.* Ithaca, NY: Cornell University Press.

Cameron, M. (2010). Faculty tenure in academe: The evolution, benefits and implications of an important tradition. *Journal of Student Affairs at New York University, 5*, 1–11. Retrieved from http://steinhardt.nyu.edu/scmsAdmin/media/users/lh62/CameronJoSA_.pdf

Curtis, J., & Jacobe, M. (2006). *AAUP contingent faculty index 2006.* Washington, DC: American Association of University Professors. Retrieved from https://www.aaup.org/sites/default/files/files/AAUPContingentFacultyIndex2006.pdf

Dunn, S. (2014). In hindsight: Former PhD students reflect on why they jumped ship. *The Chronicle of Higher Education.* Retrieved from https://chroniclevitae.com/news/445-in-hindsight-former-ph-d-students-reflect-on-why-they-jumped-ship

Ehrenberg, Ronald G., & Zhang, L. (2005). Do tenured and tenure-track faculty matter? *Journal of Human Resources, 40*(3), 647–659.

Farkas, D. (2016). 7 reasons why bright students drop out of grad school [Blog post]. *Finish Your Thesis With Dora.* Retrieved from https://finishyourthesis.com/drop-out/

Finkelstein, M., & Schuster, J. (2001). Assessing the silent revolution: How changing demographics are reshaping the academic profession. *AAHE Bulletin, 54*, 3–7.

Groves, R. (2013). Some thoughts on the tenure decision [Blog post]. *Georgetown University, The Provost Blog.* Retrieved from https://blog.provost.georgetown.edu/some-thoughts-on-the-tenure-decision/

Harrison, J. L. (2006). Post-tenure scholarship and its implications. *University of Florida Journal of Law and Public Policy.* Retrieved from http://scholarship.law.ufl.edu/facultypub/86

Hibel, A., & Scholtz, G. (2016). Tenure in academia, the past, present and future. *Higher Ed Jobs.* Retrieved from https://www.higheredjobs.com/higheredcareers/interviews.cfm?ID=459

Mangrum, B. (2014). The not-so-simple history of tenure. *Ethos.* Retrieved from http://www.ethosreview.org/intellectual-spaces/history-of-tenure/

National Education Association (NEA). (2015). The truth about tenure in higher education. Retrieved from http://www.nea.org/home/33067.htm

Nikolioudakis, N., Tsikliras, A. C., Somarakis, S., & Stergiou, K. I. (2015). Tenure and academic deadwood. *Ethics in Science and Environmental Politics, 15*, 87–93.

Oregon State University. (2014). *Faculty handbook: Promotion and tenure guidelines.* Retrieved from http://oregonstate.edu/admin/aa/faculty-handbook-promotion-and-tenure-guidelines

Siliciano, J. (2012). A short guide to the tenure process [Blog post]. *Cornell University.* Retrieved from https://blogs.cornell.edu/facultydevelopment/files/2016/01/Key-Facts-About-the-Tenure-Process-20152-250m4a4.pdf

Teichgraeber, R. F. (2014). Tenure matters: A historian's perspective. *Journal of Academic Freedom.* Retrieved from https://www.aaup.org/JAF5/tenure-matters-historian%E2%80%99s-perspective#.WNEMQI61tE5

University of California Berkeley. (2016). The transition from graduate student to assistant professor. Retrieved from https://career.berkeley.edu/PhDs/PhDtransition

Walden, T. (1980). Higher education: Attitudes toward tenure. *The Phi Delta Kappan, 62*(3), 216–217.

2

SCHOLARLY ACTIVITY

ELEMENTS OF SCHOLARLY ACTIVITY

1. Writing and publishing

2. Understanding travel expectations

3. Writing grants

4. Giving presentations

5. Understanding the Internal Review Board (IRB) process

Carving Out Time to Write

It may seem silly to devote part of a chapter to a discussion on "carving out time to write" an abstract or a manuscript, or even creating a presentation. However, this issue becomes very real when teaching, meetings, and service activities consume the majority of your week, leaving little time to write.

Although we (the three authors) have different approaches, we all agree that carving out time to write is a must. In this chapter, we outline several different options to do this, and you can choose to implement the approach that fits your needs at any given time. How you carve out time may change from one semester to the next, depending on your teaching assignments and other obligations.

DAVID'S EXAMPLE

I started a group called the Golden Quills. We met once a week during the academic year only (beginning in September and ending in April) for three-hour intervals. New assistant professors (who needed help on writing their research findings) worked with associate and full professors. Each professor held the other professor accountable when participating and when not participating. How much have you completed on your manuscript? Where are you going to submit the manuscript? A collateral gain from this writing group was the mentoring piece and identification of how the participants can collaborate together on projects and grants.

Benefits:

- Can hold each other accountable

- Can collaborate with other projects

- Can have others edit material

CONNIE'S EXAMPLE

I like to set aside one day a week to dedicate to my scholarly activities, including writing manuscripts, writing Internal Review Board (IRB) proposals, attending meetings for grants, and so on. I consider these days "sacred," and therefore I place them on my calendar at the beginning of the semester and block out the entire day. To avoid students' requesting assistance on those particular days, I offer other office hours throughout the week. If a colleague requests a meeting on my scholarly activity day, I politely decline and offer up another day. I get into a solid routine on my scholarly day. I also will only read and respond to emails at the end of a scholarly writing day. My thoughts are not to read emails until I am able to respond to them in detail. And, I do not work on any other items other than scholarly activities.

Benefits:

- Allows for one-day focus.

- Eliminates external distractors.

- One day for scholarship is doable.

CINDY'S EXAMPLE

For those who work better while multitasking, carving out time on a daily basis might work best. Working on abstracts and manuscripts on a daily basis can be done—for example, dedicating two hours a day. Working on scholarly activity for short periods enables you to focus on the material and complete spurts of quality writing. This type of writing time does not require rereading of material on a weekly basis (catching yourself up on where you left off in the writing). It also keeps the writing on the forefront—so that as a tenure-track faculty member you are less likely to put writing on the back burner and never get to it.

Benefits:

- Keeps writing a priority.

- Daily writing mitigates confusion as to where you left off.

- Small writing spurts may prove to be less intimidating than 8 to 10 hours of writing.

PROFESSIONAL WRITING RETREAT EXAMPLE

If none of the other examples meets your fancy, try a professional writing retreat. Typically held on a long weekend, these have been helpful for focusing energies on writing. Spending an entire weekend and concentrating on writing may prove, for some, to be more conducive to productivity. An accomplished author and editor who provide writing instruction and editorial advice should lead professional writing retreats. In addition, these experts will provide detailed information on how editorial boards work and what information you need when submitting your manuscript for review.

Benefits:

- Focusing for one weekend can be helpful to eliminate distractions.

- A writing retreat may be more realistic than other options.

- Typically facilitated by an accomplished author or editor.

- Great networking opportunities.

As you can tell, faculty have different approaches to setting time aside to write. What might be successful for one faculty member may not be the best approach for another. What is important is that you start writing and develop the habit of writing. Once you develop a habit of writing, it will become part of your routine. The following are some additional considerations when developing a writing habit:

- If you are struggling to set aside time to write, spend a few minutes and list the activities or barriers that are interfering with writing.

The night before your scholarly day, set up your workspace, including your computer, pens, and paper. Have your literature review, research articles, and so on readily available. Even have tissues, bottled water, and other necessities within reach so there is no reason to get distracted.

- Once you identify the activities or barriers, develop an action plan to minimize the activities or barriers that are interfering with writing. Revisit and modify the action plan as needed if you find the amount of time allotted for writing begins to decrease.

- Often, faculty are intimidated or experience elevated anxiety related to the writing process. This is very common. In fact, the anxiety can be so debilitating that faculty decide to drop out of tenure-track positions! Identifying the triggers of the anxiety can be helpful. For example, if worrying about others' editing your writing or if worrying about a manuscript's being rejected are triggering anxiety, it might be helpful to consult with a senior faculty member and discuss how he or she has worked through similar anxieties. It is important to note that most faculty experience some anxiety related to the writing process. It is quite understandable to experience anxiety when someone else edits your writing or when you are writing on a new or unfamiliar topic and worry about whether a manuscript will be accepted or rejected by a journal.

- Writing takes time, it is hard work, and it requires confidence. It is uncommon to find a faculty member who can sit and write a manuscript in a manner of a couple hours. In fact, for most faculty, it takes significantly longer! For example, it can take at least 8 to 12 hours just to write a three-page introduction to an article. Writing is hard work! If it were easy, everyone would be writing articles and books, right? Searching for articles, reading the literature, and determining which articles are essential to discuss related to your article can take days, even weeks, to complete. Analyzing data and discussing the results require an extensive amount of time. Finally, the process of writing and submitting manuscripts to professional journals takes confidence, and maintaining confidence can be challenging. Take the perspective that the entire writing process, from reading the literature to making editorial decisions, enhances your writing. This is much more positive than letting a negative editorial decision decrease your confidence. Specifically, it is much more helpful to your confidence if you are open to learning and improving your writing.

In summary, to be successful during the tenure probationary period, you need to diligently set aside time to conduct research and write for peer-review publications. Generally, many faculty are hired for a 10-month contract consisting of the fall and spring semesters of the academic year. Although some universities and colleges may require faculty to teach in the summer months, this is not universal. For many faculty, the summer months are the time to present research at conferences, conduct their research, and write manuscripts. It is very important to establish time for these scholarly endeavors. It is expected that tenured and tenure-track faculty will be productive, which requires working on scholarly activities during the summer months. Only you can determine how productive you need to be and how best to accomplish the tasks; however, establishing a routine will most likely help you be more organized, committed, and successful.

Travel Commitments

National and international presentations are required so that dissemination of information can take place. This is a common known requirement of tenure. One area that you need to think about is the amount of travel required to and from presentations. National and international presentations are often done in tandem with conferences or national association annual meetings. When a presentation is accepted, more than likely you will be required to register for the conference and commit to attending at least one day, maybe more. When traveling to national/international conferences, account for at least two days of travel—one day to the conference and one day for travel back home. Get things squared and covered prior to leaving, including any coverage for teaching. Prior to leaving for the presentation, have your presentation completed. If it's a poster, travel with the poster in hand. (Do not baggage-check it, because you do not want it to get lost!) If the paper is a podium presentation, make sure that you have secured a laptop and have the presentation saved on a flash drive or other mechanism for easy access.

The amount of time preparing presentations, traveling to the site, and networking with peers about your work (at the conferences) is a true time commitment. However, the time will reap its benefits through developing professional connections and through dissemination of material.

When traveling, do not plan on "keeping caught up" with grading and work from home. Often, you will be able to find some time after the presentation when you can go back to the hotel room, open up the laptop, and start answering emails. There also may be some time between conference sessions when you can grade a few assignments to avoid getting too far behind. However, there are occasions when the conference schedule is so rigorous that "keeping caught up" is not possible. Therefore, you need some sort of contingency plan for getting caught up when returning to the university. For example, if you have three days out of the office—one to travel to the conference, the second one for the presentation itself, and a third day to travel back from the conference—this time and the work that has accumulated will have to be caught up at home.

Publishing Expectations

Universities with a Carnegie Doctoral classification are more likely to require faculty to demonstrate the ability to publish in top-tier journals within their fields prior to being granted promotion and tenure. Specifically, high-ranking research-intensive universities equate prestige and their ability to obtain external funding with faculty who are publishing in top-tier journals. Prior to accepting a tenure-line position, it would behoove you to investigate how the college or university is classified.

The idea is that faculty who are able to demonstrate high levels of scholarly productivity, publish in high-quality journals, and are able to obtain external funding early in their careers are more likely to maintain high levels of productivity after being granted promotion and tenure.

Such expectations, predominately at universities with a Carnegie Doctoral classification, can result in high levels of stress among assistant professors. As a result, many beginning faculty, regardless of the university's classification, are intimidated about the publication process and become victims of the publish-or-perish ideology that is often prevalent among institutions in higher education.

However, the publication process does not have to be burdensome or intimidating. First, it is important to make the correct career decision. Prior to deciding to pursue a career in higher education, it is important for individuals to conduct self-evaluations focused on their own strengths and weaknesses related to research.

If an individual enjoys solving problems, reading published research studies, writing, collecting data, computing statistics, and analyzing data, there is a potential fit for academic positions that require extensive research. In contrast, if an individual dislikes writing, avoids reading published research, does not enjoy collaborating with others, has difficulties accepting constructive criticism, or wants immediate decisions on submitted work, pursuing a career that requires extensive research most likely is not a good decision.

CHARACTERISTICS OF SOMEONE WHO ENJOYS RESEARCH

Faculty accept positions in higher education for a variety of reasons. Some enjoy teaching, service-related activities, and developing policy, while others enjoy conducting research. Also, while most faculty exceed in the areas of teaching and service, more faculty tend to struggle with conducting high-quality research and demonstrating high levels of scholarly productivity. Gaining an understanding of the traits of someone who enjoys conducting research can help you determine whether you are a good fit for an institution with high research expectations. The following provides some characteristics of someone who enjoys research:

- Finds solving complex problems interesting

- Likes answering questions that can affect clinical practice

- Can spend hours writing and revising manuscripts

- Does not consider it a chore to read published research

- Finds collecting data interesting

- Has the ability to synthesize and analyze data

- Has the patience to conduct research that may take months or even years to complete

- Enjoys collaborating with others

- Is able to withstand constructive criticism

- Has a never-give-up attitude

If you enjoy research (or even if you are forcing yourself to conduct research), it is important to identify your research strengths and learn effective strategies to address your weaknesses. For example, the majority of research studies require some type of statistical analyses; however, although most researchers have basic knowledge of statistics, most researchers are not expert statisticians. Therefore, recognizing when to consult with a statistician or, more importantly, learning when to turn over the statistical analysis to a statistician is an important skill.

A faculty member who struggles with writing a results section but enjoys reading the published literature and writing introductions and discussion sections of manuscripts may decide to collaborate with another researcher who enjoys writing results sections of manuscripts. Many faculty think they have to conduct research on their own or are often hesitant to approach other faculty with hopes of developing collaborative research projects. Senior faculty know what many beginning faculty have not learned: All researchers have strengths and weaknesses when it comes to conducting research and publishing. They also have learned that collaboration increases the quality of research and, as a result, increases the faculty member's chances of research being accepted for publication.

Why Publishing Can Be Challenging

It is not uncommon for faculty to struggle the first two or three years in publishing research. In fact, the faculty member who publishes one to two publications per year from year one is the exception. It is more common for faculty to struggle the first two or three years as they acclimate to the demands of higher education and learn to balance teaching, research, and service activities.

Faculty struggle with publishing for a variety of reasons. However, some of the more common reasons are listed here:

- Poor writing (e.g., too many spelling and grammar errors, verb-tense errors)

- Poor data (e.g., small sample size and not enough power, too many participants missing data, samples not reflective of the population the study is generalizing to, etc.)

- Submits to the wrong journals (e.g., manuscript does not align with the scope or mission of the journal, submits only to journals with high rejection rates)

- Poorly designed research studies (e.g., methodology issues, unclear procedures, confounds not accounted for, etc.)

- Does not revise and resubmit manuscripts if rejected

- Does not follow required manuscript format style (e.g., APA style)

- Becomes discouraged and gives up

- Does not accept constructive feedback from journal editors

- Does not revise research to address issues raised by journal reviewers—repeats same methodological errors over and over

- Does not discuss current research in manuscript (e.g., sources are dated, manuscript fails to recognize seminal work in the field, theoretical framework for the study is lacking, etc.)

All the aforementioned issues can slow the scholarly productivity of faculty during the first two or three years. However, the learning curve on how to conduct research, where to submit manuscripts for publication, and how to revise and resubmit manuscripts that have been rejected is fairly sharp. To be blunt, most faculty figure it out! In part, the key is perseverance and maintaining a positive attitude. However, for faculty who continue to struggle with productivity, the following sidebar provides several suggestions on how to increase and maintain scholarly productivity.

SUGGESTIONS ON HOW TO INCREASE SCHOLARLY PRODUCTIVITY

- ❑ Set aside four to six hours each week specifically for writing, and protect this time.

- ❑ Join a writing group that meets at least once a week, and protect this time.

- ❑ Set aside two to three days for writing after the semester is over, and protect this time.

- ❑ Find a location that is free from distractions or temptations (e.g., visiting with a colleague, putting laundry in the washing machine, children wanting assistance with homework, etc.) when writing.

- ❑ Turn off your cell phone when writing.

- ❑ Do not log into your email on the days you set aside for writing.

- ❑ Ask a senior faculty member to read and provide constructive feedback on manuscripts prior to submitting them to journals for possible publication.

- ❑ Have no more than two or three manuscripts in preparation at any one time.

- ❑ Always have at least one manuscript under review by a journal.

- ❑ Revise and resubmit manuscripts that have been rejected or are rejected with the option of resubmission within 30 days.

- ❑ Develop two to three collaborative research projects with other faculty.

- ❑ Gain input from senior faculty on possible publication outlets and where you might submit manuscripts for possible publication.

- ❑ Avoid writing external grants unless external funding is a requirement for promotion and tenure.

- ❑ Write and apply for internal grants to support your research.

- ❑ Know when to move on with a manuscript or research project. Not all manuscripts are accepted for publication, and not all research projects result in publishable data.

❑ Effectively use research and graduate assistants.

❑ Run all your work through software programs that check for plagiarism.

❑ Start the reference list and complete full references as you write.

❑ Have research reviews primarily completed prior to sitting and starting to write.

❑ Turn conference presentations into manuscripts you can submit to journals for possible publication.

❑ Submit a proposal to journals you publish in that accept proposals for special issues.

Publications, Presentations, and Grants

Faculty often ask whether publications, presentations, or grants are more important when pursing promotion and tenure. For faculty pursuing promotion and tenure from assistant to associate, it is generally agreed that publications carry more weight than presentations or grants (at most institutions). However, it is important for faculty to be familiar with the promotion and tenure requirements for their departments, colleges, and universities. Generally, most institutions are looking for faculty to publish a minimum of one manuscript per year in refereed journals with fairly low acceptance rates (10% to 20%). At some universities with a Carnegie Doctoral classification, the minimum number of refereed journal publications may range as high as two or more per year! If this is the case, it is easy to see that publications are given higher consideration during promotion and tenure deliberations.

So, should faculty present papers and posters at national/international conferences? Absolutely! Presentations at conferences often lead to other publications or collaborative opportunities, while also increasing the national/international visibility of the institution. In addition, the majority of institutions require that the presentations be peer-refereed prior to being accepted for presentation.

How important are presentations to department and college promotion and tenure (P&T) committees when making promotion and tenure recommendations? In short, they are considered but do not carry the same weight as publications. Regardless, most universities require the minimum of one to two national/international presentations per year. The faculty member who is publishing fewer than one manuscript per year on average but has a large number of presentations (three or more a year) is likely to receive a negative promotion and tenure decision, especially if the faculty member is at a university with a Carnegie Doctoral classification.

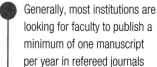 Generally, most institutions are looking for faculty to publish a minimum of one manuscript per year in refereed journals with fairly low acceptance rates (10% to 20%).

Aside from the expense of traveling and presenting at a large number of conferences (most universities have limited travel funds, so the faculty member incurs the costs), preparing and presenting at a large number of conferences takes time away from writing and publishing. In short, the faculty member's time would be better spent focusing on writing, and most promotion and tenure committees are likely to make the recommendation to present less and write more!

A few final comments related to presentations: Most universities place little to no weight on presentations at state and regional professional meetings. In fact, presentations at state and regional meetings would be better located under professional service activities within the vitae.

To gain the most from presentations, due to the preparation and travel time involved, take the perspective that presentations are not complete until they have been turned into a manuscript that can be submitted for publication. Many presentations just need some additional reformatting or minimal writing to prepare them for submission. With this approach, faculty can meet both the presentation and publication requirements within a given year.

Publishing to Online and Open-Access Journals

Over the last 10 years, there has been a substantial increase in open-access electronic journals. *Open access* refers to manuscripts that are published electronically on the Internet and are available to anyone. Many of the open-access journals are pay journals. However, there are also journals that still print hard copies that are pay journals. A *pay journal* is defined as a journal that requires authors to pay some type of fee at time of submission, prior to the manuscript's being sent out to reviewers and/or after the manuscript has been accepted. These fees typically are charged to cover printing, typesetting (e.g., editing, reformatting), production, mailing, and other editorial administrative costs. Obviously, the printing and typesetting costs are related mostly to hard-copy journals. Overall, the number of hard-copy journals is slowly decreasing, whereas the number of electronic, open-access journals is growing rapidly.

It is fairly easy to find open-access online journals in nursing that are willing to review submitted manuscripts, send them out for blind review, and accept manuscripts for publication while at the same time charging publication fees. Although there are legitimate online journals, there are also thousands of predatory journals waiting to take researchers' money. A *predatory journal* accepts publication fees without providing any editorial services (e.g., sending the manuscript out for review, editing, publishing, etc.). Predatory journals often require payment of fees at the time of submission. However, some predatory journals indicate that once a manuscript is accepted for publication, the author then needs to pay a fee to help cover the publication costs. Other predatory journals charge several small fees at different stages of the editorial process, as the manuscript supposedly is being reviewed and processed for publication. These fees can range from fairly small amounts (e.g., $100 to $300) to large amounts (e.g., $1000 to more than $5000).

Predatory journals are becoming fairly sophisticated and can give the appearance of being legitimate journals; therefore, faculty considering submitting a manuscript to an open-access online journal should research the journal's history prior to submitting a manuscript.

> The Scholarly Open Access website (https://scholarlyoa.com/publishers/) provides Beall's List of potential, possible, or probable predatory scholarly open-access publishers. This list is routinely updated.

There are legitimate journals, online journals, and open-access journals to which faculty can submit manuscripts for possible publication. Several of these journals are as rigorous (e.g., editor is well known in the field, editorial board consists of major researchers in the field, all manuscripts receive a double-blind review, etc.) as well-established printed journals. In fact, many of the well-established printed journals are moving toward or are now electronic journals (some require a fee or journal subscription to access publications). These online journals and open-access online journals should be considered legitimate publication outlets.

Should faculty submit manuscripts to pay journals, even if they are legitimate? Well, it depends! Some universities frown on the idea of faculty's submitting and publishing manuscripts to pay journals, even if the journals are legitimate and use a double-blind review process.

It is important to review the department, college, and university promotion and tenure documents to determine whether publishing in pay journals is permissible. However, more than likely, the issue of pay journals is not addressed. Therefore, it is recommended that faculty discuss submitting and publishing in pay journals with the department chair and the chair of the P&T committee. If given the green light to publish in pay journals, it is important to gain approval in writing (e.g., a quick email indicating it is fine to publish in pay journals).

When publishing in pay journals, it is important to consider their acceptance rates. Typically, pay journals have higher acceptance rates (more than 40%) compared to nonpay journals. If the institution is more focused on faculty publishing and places minimal weight on acceptance rates, publishing in a pay journal may make sense, if a faculty member is willing to pay the publication fee. It is important to note that most universities will not cover or reimburse faculty for publication fees related to pay journals. If the university places significant weight on journals' acceptance rates, then faculty should be judicious when deciding to publish in pay journals.

Considering the Journal's Impact Factor

A journal's *impact factor* (IF) is the average number of times other authors cite articles published in that journal. For example, an IF of 2.0 for a nursing journal indicates that, on average, authors publishing manuscripts in other journals cited articles in the nursing journal an average of two times over the past year. Specifically, if the nursing journal published 40 manuscripts during 2016, and during the 2017 calendar year authors cited manuscripts 80 times that were published in the nursing journal during 2016, the IF (80 divided by 40 = 2.0) would be 2.0. Because the IF is an average, some manuscripts published in the nursing journal during 2016 could have been cited more than twice, whereas other articles may not have been cited at all.

Why are journal IFs important to authors and promotion and tenure? Many universities with a Carnegie Doctoral classification place significant weight on journal IFs when making promotion and tenure decisions. Although there is an emphasis on scholarly productivity, many universities with a Carnegie Doctoral classification also want faculty to publish in prestigious journals. In short, they like it when their faculty are publishing in journals that faculty at other institutions are reading and citing. Their faculty are conducting meaningful and impactful research that others are citing.

> Nursing journals with high IFs are generally viewed as making a more significant contribution to the field compared to journals with lower IFs. A journal with an IF of 2.5 or higher is generally viewed as making a significant impact on the field.

At some institutions, the focus is not on quantity but on quality. The institution would rather faculty conduct high-quality research that is published in journals with low acceptance rates and high IFs. Consequently, the environment supports research that may take years to publish.

Again, faculty are encouraged to read the department, college, and university promotion and tenure documents to determine a university's requirements, if any, related to publishing in journals with high IFs. However, it is fairly common for institutions not to address IF in department, college, and university promotion and tenure documents. That said, there can sometimes be unwritten rules that IFs need to be reported along with acceptance/rejection rates when faculty submit materials for review by the various promotion and tenure committees. It is better to gain an understanding of the expectations for reporting IFs and acceptance rates early, as it will help determine the type of journals faculty submit manuscripts to for possible publication.

Determining Order of Authorship

Order of authorship is typically determined by the amount of contribution each author makes. Authors make decisions and agree on order of authorship based on a variety of approaches and reasons. Not all follow ethical standards or professional guidelines. Also, the approaches used by different disciplines vary widely. The following are some of the more common reasons authors have used to determine order of authorship:

- The author who spent the most time writing and editing the manuscript is the first author.

- The most challenging section to write was the introduction, so it is decided that the first author should be the one who wrote the introduction.

- The researcher who came up with the idea to develop the study is the first author.

- Two authors who collaborate together on research decide to rotate first authorship regardless of who contributes the most to writing an article.

- Senior faculty pressure junior faculty to list the senior faculty as first author, even if the junior faculty wrote the majority of the manuscript.

- One faculty is on an editorial board, so to increase the chances that the manuscript is accepted, the faculty member on the editorial board is listed as the first author.

- The faculty member allows another faculty to use a large dataset with the agreement that he or she be listed as the first author.

- The faculty member who wrote the grant and obtained funding is the first author on all research published.

- A graduate student should not be listed first, because he or she is being paid to write as part of the graduate assistantship.

- The faculty member is pursuing promotion and tenure and has not senior-authored a manuscript, so he or she needs to be the first author.

Obviously, many of these reasons likely violate ethical practice and are inconsistent with professional standards within the field of nursing. However, they illustrate how authorship, especially first authorship, is sometimes decided. The majority of time, faculty decide order of authorship based on the amount of contribution each researcher (even graduate students collaborating on research) makes toward developing and implementing a study and writing the manuscript, which is consistent with professional guidelines.

When several researchers working on the same study make similar contributions, most of the time an amicable decision is made related to the order of authorship. When faculty decide on the order of authorship prior to starting to write a manuscript, and one faculty member ends up contributing more to the manuscript than the predetermined first author, it can result in resentment by the faculty member who did a higher percentage of the writing. Therefore, it is critical to agree that in the end, the faculty member who contributes the most to writing the manuscript will be the first author.

How important is it for faculty to demonstrate senior authorship when publishing? At some universities with a Carnegie Doctoral classification, it is very important to demonstrate the ability to publish research as the first author. In fact, at many institutions, it would be difficult for a faculty member to be promoted and tenured with no senior authorships. More likely, the expectation would be to demonstrate senior authorship on at least one, and up to three, publications. At more prestigious universities, there can be significant pressure for faculty to be the first author on a majority of their publications.

At some institutions, faculty are required to describe their contribution (e.g., wrote introduction, conducted data analysis, wrote the results section, and so on) and/or indicate the percentage of their contribution for every manuscript published in a professional journal, regardless of the order of authorship. Therefore, at institutions where the order of authorship is considered by P&T committees, it can result in faculty's vying for senior authorship or can lead to fewer collaborative research projects. Fortunately, many institutions encourage collaboration and do not require that the majority of publications by a faculty member be senior authored.

MANAGING AUTHORSHIP AND TENURE

A final point on the order of authorship: Although most institutions are not overly focused on faculty's demonstrating senior authorship or the order of authorship, it would be difficult for an individual to be recommended for tenure if he/she were consistently listed only as the third, fourth, or fifth author on all publications. There should be at least a few first and second authorships. Also, if a faculty member were listed as the last author on several publications, even with a couple of first or second authorships, most P&T committees would likely wonder whether the individual were just added to publications to help with tenure.

Editorial Decisions: Accepted, Rejected, or Revise

It is rare for manuscripts submitted to refereed journals to be accepted without at least minor revisions. If a manuscript is accepted with minor revisions, faculty should make the revisions and resubmit within a couple of days, if not sooner.

Manuscripts that receive a decision of rejection with an option to resubmit (reject and resubmit) should always be resubmitted. Faculty are often disappointed with a reject-and-resubmit decision; however, revising and resubmitting the manuscript greatly increases the chances it will be accepted. With reject-and-resubmit decisions, most editors provide specific timelines for resubmission. Faculty should always revise and resubmit within the specified timelines. In addition, it is essential to provide a detailed letter addressing the revisions, revisions requested by the editor, and revisions requested by the reviewers and addressing any requested revisions that were not made. If any of the requested revisions are not made, authors should provide a rationale for why they were not addressed.

The most common decision by refereed journals is rejection. It is important to remember this. The majority of refereed journals have a rejection rate of 60% to 75%, and the more prestigious journals typically have an 85% to 90% rejection rate. The odds are that a manuscript submitted for consideration by a refereed journal will be rejected. Therefore, faculty who view rejections as a learning experience and an opportunity to enhance the manuscript prior to resubmitting to another journal will fair far better compared to faculty who view the submission process negatively and react with anger. All faculty will have manuscripts rejected by professional journals—*all* faculty.

Faculty who learn to accept constructive feedback and avoid personalizing rejections will be more successful in publishing research. Unless there are fatal flaws with the study (e.g., unaccounted confounds, lack of a control group when needed, lack of generalizability of the findings, etc.), faculty should continue to revise and resubmit the manuscript to other journals.

Original Research and the Internal Review Board

During the tenure probationary process, you will be expected to conduct original research. If you did not complete a master's degree thesis or a doctoral dissertation, then you might consider working with a colleague or requesting a faculty mentor to help guide you through the process of conducting research. Research should be an exciting adventure; it's not to be feared or dreaded. Some of the first steps are to determine your area of interest, whether the topic is sustainable over a long period of time, and whether there are grant monies available to help fund your research. It's important to discuss these areas with a more experienced researcher prior to making a decision; doing so may ensure better success. There are different thoughts about establishing a line of research. Some promotion and tenure committees allow faculty to establish several lines of research that complement each other, whereas other institutions require faculty to establish a single line of research. You need to discuss this issue with your faculty mentor, department chair, and chair of the promotion and tenure committee before you make a final decision and move forward with any research.

It is important to be fully vested in whatever area of research you determine is right for you, because you will be conducting the research over the lifetime of your tenured career. There are many types of research that fall in the categories of quantitative and qualitative methodology, so understanding both methods is also critical to your success. Additionally, it is necessary to gain insight into what original research is and why is it important during the tenure probationary period.

Newton (2016) describes several key elements to help identify original research:

1. Original research is generally the report written by the researcher(s) who conducted the study.

2. The hypothesis and the research question(s) are identified.

3. There is a detailed methods section.

4. The results or findings from the research are described.

5. Conclusions based on the evidence and implications for the future are acknowledged.

6. There is an detailed reference list.

Majumder (2015) describes original research as the main source of scientific research from original studies found in the published literature. The information submitted must be written by the researcher who conducted the study. Inexperienced researchers might believe that a negative finding is not valid or publishable, but that is not true. Negative findings are of value and should be submitted in a manuscript for possible publication (Majumder, 2015). It is very important that the researcher conduct studies ethically and legally, following established protocol.

Understanding the Internal Review Board Process

The IRB process is required for research conducted in the United States and most of the world. The IRB process is rigorous and necessary to protect all individuals and animals from undue physical and emotional harm. "The purpose of IRB review is to assure, both in advance and by periodic review, that appropriate steps are taken to protect the rights and welfare of humans participating as subjects in the research. To accomplish this purpose, IRBs use a group process to review research protocols and related materials (e.g., informed consent documents and investigator brochures) to ensure protection of the rights and welfare of human subjects of research" (fda.gov, 2016).

Navigating Through the Internal Review Board Process

After you have identified a line or lines of research you want to study, it is important that you review and understand the IRB process in the institution where you will be conducting your research. Failure to comply with IRB rules and regulations might jeopardize not only your study but also your reputation as a researcher. All universities in the United States have IRB protocols and committees that are present to protect your rights as a researcher as well as the rights of the research participants. Navigating though the IRB process might seem like an arduous task, but it is necessary.

The first step in the IRB process is to complete the Collaborative Institutional Training Initiative (CITI) training. The mission of the CITI training is

> *[to] promote the public's trust in the research enterprise by providing high quality, peer reviewed, web based, research education materials to enhance the integrity and professionalism of investigators and staff conducting research.* (Citiprogram.org, 2016)

CITI training is important, because it is necessary to learn the historical evolution of the safeguards for human subjects and significant historical unethical events that were instrumental in the creation of informed consents and regulatory limitations to research. The CITI training course is made up of two sections: Biomedical and Social-Behavioral-Education (SBE) and a series of Additional Modules of Interest (citiprogram.org, 2016). There are additional courses for individuals seeking positions on IRB boards or committees or who are seeking to learn more about the roles and responsibilities of the IRB administrators. After you have completed the CITI training and received a certificate of completion, it is important to retain the certificate.

It is important to note that each institution will likely have different requirements related to CITI training. Therefore, it is essential to become familiar with your institution's IRB guidelines. In addition, different disciplines and agencies are likely to have additional IRB policies and procedures that may need to be addressed prior to your starting research.

The IRB submission process for full or expedited review should include the following:

1. The purpose of the study and the procedures that will be taken

2. The anticipated risks and benefits to the study participants

3. What safeguards will be taken to protect the study participants

4. Procedures outlining how study participants are obtained

5. A detailed informed consent (BSU.edu, 2016; Colgate University, n.d.)

After you submit the required documents to the institution's IRB, you will receive notification that the documents have been submitted and are undergoing review. If it is determined that there is minimal risk to your participants, most likely an exempt status will be issued; otherwise, the submission will undergo a full board review prior to a final decision. As the researcher, you are responsible for all IRB documentation and regulation before, during, and after your study. When your study is complete, you are required to submit a final report summarizing your study and the results to the IRB; then, a notification of study closure will be issued.

Maintaining Integrity in Research

As a researcher, you are expected to maintain high ethical and professional standards. It is important that publishers and the public trust your work. Mulvey (2015) explains that universities create ethical challenges for researchers simply by the nature of the "publish-or-perish" atmosphere and pressure placed on tenured and tenure-track faculty with regard to scholarly productivity as applied to recruitment, retention, tenure, and research grants. Mulvey states, "Those engaged in scientific research assume an extraordinary obligation to fellow researchers, and the world in general. They must observe accepted protocols associated with any confidential data or techniques derived under a consulting contract, abide by the regulations of their home institutions, and at the same time make their fellow researchers and the world in general aware of their findings and conclusions. It is a balancing act" (479).

The term *science* usually refers to this method and to the organized body of information that has been derived from using this logical approach to thinking and investigation. Rational, open-ended, honest inquiry is the means by which science unravels the truth. Hence, science has been called "a candle in the dark" (Harris, 2011). Researchers are revered for revealing the truth, but when trust is broken, the results can have dire consequences (Sagan, 1996). Academic dishonesty hurts everyone, so it is the responsibility of every faculty conducting research to adhere to the highest ethical standards and practices to ensure the integrity of scientific research.

PLAGIARISM

Most faculty understand that plagiarism can result in termination and/or the denial of promotion and tenure. Also, most faculty understand that the intentional use of other authored work and claiming it as their own without appropriately citing the work is considered plagiarism. However, faculty often unintentionally commit plagiarism. Faculty need to be careful when copying or even paraphrasing content found on the Internet. Many websites copy content from other web pages or sources without citing the original source.

Self-plagiarism also is a concept many faculty do not understand. Many faculty believe that because they worked on and published a manuscript, they own the material that was published. However, most journals require authors to sign a copyright form giving proprietary ownership of all content to the publisher. Faculty who include portions of the published article within future manuscripts are actually plagiarizing. For example, an individual who uses the same language to describe the participants and procedures in another study using the same data is actually committing plagiarism. The faculty member needs to rewrite the participants and procedures section or paraphrase and cite the original source, even if he or she is citing his or her own publication.

Chapter Checkup

❏ Do I have an appreciation and understanding of the time commitment for scholarly activity, including writing manuscripts and traveling to present?

❏ Do I understand the publishing expectations at my institution?

❏ Do I possess the characteristics of someone who enjoys conducting research?

❏ Do I have a clear understanding of the challenges of getting published, and do I have a plan to avoid these pitfalls?

❏ Do I have a plan to implement positive strategies to increase my own scholarly productivity?

❑ Do I understand the different weights that my own institution places on publications, presentations, and grants with regard to the P&T process?

❑ Do I have a clear understanding of the difference in online and open-access journals and how my institution views each of these publishing options?

❑ Do I possess the knowledge of what a journal's IF is and what my institution's expectations are related to IFs?

❑ Do I understand the various ways authorship is determined?

❑ Do I understand the reason for IRB and how to navigate through the IRB process, including the reasons for CITI training?

References

Ball State University (BSU). (2016). Research integrity. Retrieved from http://cms. bsu.edu/about/administrativeoffices/researchintegrity/humansubjects/preparing-humansubjectsproposal

Citiprogram.org. (2016). Collaborative Institutional Training Initiative at the University of Miami. *CITI Program.* Retrieved from https://www.citiprogram.org/index. cfm?pageID=30

Colgate University. (n.d.). General guidelines for IRB proposal. Retrieved from http://www.colgate.edu/academics/departments-and-programs/psychology/ institutional-review-board/general-guidelines

Food and Drug Administration (FDA). (2016). Institutional review boards frequently asked questions–Information sheet. *U.S. Food and Drug Administration. Department of Health and Human Services.* Retrieved from http://www.fda.gov/ RegulatoryInformation/Guidances/ucm126420.htm

Harris, S. (2011). *The moral landscape: How science can determine human values.* London, U.K.: Transworld Digital [Kindle edition, location 137 of 7423].

Majumder, K. (2015). A young researcher's guide to writing an original research article. *Editage.com.* Retrieved from http://www.editage.com/insights/a-young-researchers-guide-to-writing-an-original-research-article

Mulvey, G. J. (2015). Ethics in research. *American Meteorological Society.* doi:10.1175/BAMS-D-13-00272.1

Newton, L. (2016). What is original research? *University of North Florida. Thomas G. Carpenter Library.* Retrieved from http://libguides.unf.edu/originalresearch

Sagan C. (1996). *The demon-haunted world: Science as a candle in the dark.* New York, NY: Ballantine Books.

3

SERVICE

ELEMENTS OF SERVICE

1. Ensures faculty are participating in their "fair share" of university committees

2. Allows faculty to share their expertise at professional levels

3. Provides faculty different options to meet their service requirements

4. Encourages and requires faculty to give back to their individual professions

---

An important part of successfully making tenure is fulfilling the service requirements set forth by your institution. Professional service typically involves, but isn't limited to, membership on department, college, and university committees; journal editorial advisory boards; professional committees; and so on. In fact, service can be broken into several areas, all of which are covered in this chapter:

- National professional service
- University service
- Clinical-related professional service
- Community service

National Professional Service

Professional service is a requirement at most colleges and universities. Therefore, faculty cannot ignore service and must consider service important when pursuing promotion and tenure.

Compared to research and teaching requirements, the requirements for service often tend to be more vague. In fact, most promotion and tenure documents refer to service but do not provide specific criteria or outline service requirements. Major universities often have different service expectations than two- and four-year colleges. For example, universities with a Carnegie Doctoral classification often expect national service, whereas two- and four-year colleges often focus on state and regional service activities.

Faculty at prestigious universities often become involved in national associations by serving on committees, chairing committees, and becoming officers (e.g., president, secretary, vice president, and so on). Serving on editorial boards or having positions as an associate editor or editor of major journals also is common. Faculty also serve as site visitors for accrediting bodies and/or licensing boards, which often requires extensive travel or meetings. Although some universities do not specifically indicate in promotion and tenure documents the particular types of service mentioned here, it's often an unwritten expectation that faculty must begin to show national service prior to being granted promotion and tenure. Faculty pursuing promotion from associate to full professor almost always must demonstrate extensive service at the national level, especially at universities with a Carnegie Doctoral classification.

Compared to national service activities, most major universities place minimal weight on state and regional service when making promotion and tenure decisions. The opposite is true for two- and four-year colleges, which often have minimal, if any, national service expectations but typically encourage service at the state and regional levels. Faculty at smaller universities who demonstrate service at the national level often stand out among their peers and can actually receive merit and promotion solely based on their national service activities.

Interestingly, many universities do not provide travel support for the sole purpose of faculty participation in national service activities. Faculty, however, are fairly creative and often will submit a poster, paper, or symposium at major conferences (which are often paid for by universities) and while at the conference attend committee meetings. Also, some national associations and organizations cover some of the travel costs for officers to attend meetings, which helps reduce faculty costs.

Faculty should be selective about the types of national service activities they pursue. In short, it can become very expensive to serve on several national committees if a faculty member has to pay for hotel, travel, and food expenses out of pocket.

Attending a national conference enables you to meet two different tenure require-ments (scholarly activity and service). For example, when you're presenting at a national conference, also volunteer to be a moderator at one of the breakout sessions. As a session moderator, you are providing a service. A collateral gain is that it enables you to begin networking within the professional association or organization.

University Service

Service at the department, college, and university levels is also expected at most universities. The majority of faculty start demon-strating service at the department level and gradually increase service activities at the college and university levels. It is uncommon for first-year faculty to chair university committees; they also are more likely to serve on committees for a couple of years before starting to chair. There typically are a large number of committees faculty can serve on, even as first-year faculty. Therefore, many department chairs tend to be protective of first- and second-year faculty and encourage them to limit the number of committees they serve on.

BE SELECTIVE, AND DON'T OVERCOMMIT

It is important to not overcommit time to service, especially to committees, during the first five to six years after starting a tenure-track position. Faculty often underestimate the time commitment of committee work. Some commit-tees meet only a couple of times each semester, whereas other committees might meet weekly. A faculty member serving on five or six committees that tend to meet six to eight times per semester can quickly lose 30 to 48 hours per semester that could be used to write a manuscript. It's also important to consider outside committee work that takes time away from writing. Preparing for meetings can actually take several hours, especially for national commit-tees. For national committees, travel also can easily result in faculty's losing several days of quality writing time. It is helpful to consider the following issues when deciding which committees to serve on:

- How often and when does the committee meet?

- Does the committee require extensive preparation prior to each meeting? For example, serving on an institution's Internal Review Board (IRB) committee will require an extensive amount of preparation compared to serving on the college travel committee, which focuses on approving funding to support faculty travel to conferences.

- Does the committee have several subcommittees, which will require additional meetings and preparation?

- Will you be expected to chair the committee at some point?

- Committees focused on accreditation often require an extensive amount of work and have several work groups focused on addressing each accreditation standard, resulting in significant time commitments.

- Many regional and state-level committees meet during the weekend due to the nonacademic members' having nine-to-five jobs. Serving on these committees often requires you give up four to six Saturdays a year. Although serving on regional and state-level committees is a great way to connect with other professionals locally, it also is important to balance professional and family commitments. Using weekends to serve on professional committees greatly decreases time spent with family and friends.

- Prior to agreeing to serve on national committees, it is helpful to know whether all their meetings require you to participate in person or whether you can participate in some of the meetings via Skype, FaceTime, or phone conferencing.

- Serving on alumni councils also can require you to attend evening and weekend alumni functions.

In summary, committee service, whether at the national, state, regional, or university level, can become quite time-consuming. Therefore, faculty should be highly selective about the types of committees they agree to serve on. Faculty should strive to demonstrate a balance of work across national, state, regional, and university committees. There should be enough service across all levels to demonstrate a commitment to service without causing service to significantly affect teaching or scholarly productivity.

Although faculty need to demonstrate service on department, college, and university committees, serving on a large number of committees does not lead to a positive promotion and tenure decision at doctoral-level institutions. At non-doctoral-level institutions, where there is less pressure to publish, there can be higher service expectations.

Clinical-Related Professional Service

At many institutions, outside professional clinical service or consultation is expected. Although many universities limit the amount of outside (outside the university) paid professional service (e.g., no more than 8 hours per week is allowed), they also expect nursing faculty to stay current in their specialty areas. In fact, in some states, for nurses to maintain their licenses, they are required to complete a minimum number of clinical hours per month. For example, a faculty member who teaches medical-surgical courses might work one day per week in a medical-surgical unit at a hospital to stay current with advancements in the field. Although listing medical-surgical work as professional service is important, it is highly unlikely that a promotion and tenure committee would place much weight on this type of service when making tenure decisions at most major universities. It might carry more weight at two- and four-year colleges, though.

As you consider outside professional clinical service, keep these points in mind: It is important to review the university handbook policy related to outside paid-work activities. Some universities might have strict limitations on any outside paid work. Also, some universities might not classify outside paid work as service and not allow it to be considered as part of promotion and tenure decisions.

SERVICE PROGRESSION

An example of service progression may look like this:

Year 1: One department committee and required clinical service and participating in professional organization at state or national level.

Year 2: As above, and add one college committee.

Year 3: As above, and add chairing the college committee as well as participating in one editorial board (in your area of expertise).

Year 4: As above, and add university committee.

Year 5: As above, and add chairing university committee and consider being member of thesis or dissertation committee.

Year 6: As above, and add chairing thesis or dissertation committee.

Year 7: As above, and add national leadership chair of professional organization.

The following table shows a typical schedule.

Sunday	Monday	Tuesday	Wednesday	Thursday	Friday	Saturday
	Teaching	Outside Paid Service Activity	Teaching	Clinic	Scholarly Activities	
	Teaching	Outside Paid Service Activity	Teaching	Clinic	Scholarly Activities	
	Teaching	Outside Paid Service Activity	Teaching	Clinic	Scholarly Activities	
	Office Hours	Outside Paid Service Activity	Office Hours	Clinic	Scholarly Activities	
Prep for Teaching	Prep for Meeting	Outside Paid Service Activity		Admission and Progression Meeting (department service)	Scholarly Activities	
Prep for Teaching	Student Advisory Group (college service)	Outside Paid Service Activity			Scholarly Activities	

Here are some practical points to consider prior to committing to professional service:

- Committing to working at a hospital, physician's office, or other healthcare setting is a big decision. Often, the added stress of working with patients can leave you emotionally and physically exhausted and require a couple of days to recover, therefore affecting your responsibilities within the academic setting. If you notice you are too exhausted to fulfill your academic responsibilities, address it immediately.

- If you pursue outside work, it will be important to set limits on the day(s) and hours per week you will work and to make sure your employer is clear on the day(s) and hours you will work each week. It is not uncommon for employers to attempt to increase your hours and to attempt to have you fill in other days of the week. Set limits, and stick to your original agreement.

- If you find that work related to your professional service activities is having to be completed at home in the evenings or during the weekends, take steps to avoid bringing the work home. The work at home will increase the likelihood of your burning out and decrease your level of scholarly productivity.

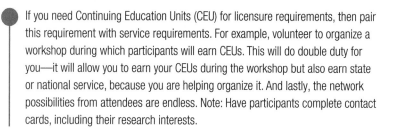

If you need Continuing Education Units (CEU) for licensure requirements, then pair this requirement with service requirements. For example, volunteer to organize a workshop during which participants will earn CEUs. This will do double duty for you—it will allow you to earn your CEUs during the workshop but also earn state or national service, because you are helping organize it. And lastly, the network possibilities from attendees are endless. Note: Have participants complete contact cards, including their research interests.

Master's and Doctoral Thesis Committees

Faculty working in departments that offer master's or doctoral degrees may also be expected to serve on and chair thesis committees. Although serving on a thesis committee is much less time-consuming than chairing a thesis committee, they both require significant time commitments. Agreeing to serve on more than one or two thesis committees per year, or agreeing to chair more than one thesis committee per year, quickly consumes a large number of hours. Even if a faculty member agrees to serve on or chair one thesis committee per year, it is not uncommon for several graduate students to need continuous advisement for two or more years until their theses are completed and defended. In addition, serving as the chair often can lead to presentations and publications after the thesis has been completed.

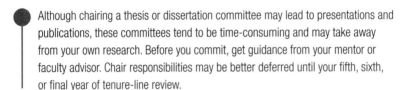

Although chairing a thesis or dissertation committee may lead to presentations and publications, these committees tend to be time-consuming and may take away from your own research. Before you commit, get guidance from your mentor or faculty advisor. Chair responsibilities may be better deferred until your fifth, sixth, or final year of tenure-line review.

Promotion and Tenure Committee

It might seem unusual for a nontenured faculty member to serve on a promotion and tenure committee, but some institutions actually allow or even encourage participation. The view is that nontenured faculty who serve on the promotion and tenure committee gain insight related to the expectations of promotion and tenure. The majority of institutions, however, do not allow nontenured faculty to serve on promotion and tenure committees.

Serving on a promotion and tenure committee as a nontenured assistant professor can be quite intimidating, especially if the committee includes senior faculty. It also can be fairly awkward for an assistant professor to have to step out while the committee conducts deliberations regarding his/her progress toward tenure and then have to step back into the meeting. Therefore, if a university allows nontenured faculty to serve on promotion and tenure committees, it might be best to avoid serving on this committee. Promotion and tenure is stressful enough without becoming part of the decision-making process for others.

Community Service

Many faculty confuse professional service with community service. *Professional service*, as discussed previously, is related to the profession of nursing (e.g., national committees, serving as a site visitor, serving as grant reviewer, and so on) or the university. *Community service* is considered volunteer work that may or may not be related to your professional identity as a nurse or faculty member at the university. For example, serving as secretary on a church committee, chairing the parent-teacher-student organization at a local school, or donating time at the local soup kitchen is community service. In short, at most institutions, community service is not considered with regard to promotion and tenure decisions. However, some small colleges or religious-affiliated universities might have expectations related to community service and, therefore, consider community service when making promotion and tenure decisions. For the majority of institutions, it is better not to list community service on the vitae, especially when professional service is the primary requirement for promotion and tenure.

SUGGESTIONS TO INCREASE SERVICE

❑ Begin your second-year focus on serving on at least one or two departmental committees.

❑ During years 3 to 7, focus on serving on at least one college committee and one university committee per year.

❑ Avoid chairing a departmental committee until after your third year.

❑ Avoid chairing a college or university committee until after your fourth year.

❑ During years 1 to 3, start providing ad hoc reviews for journals specific to your field.

❑ After your third year, begin to request membership on one to two editorial boards to which you have been providing ad hoc reviews over the last two years.

❑ As you begin to present at professional conferences during years 1 and 2, start attending meetings (e.g., board meetings, interest groups, open meetings with journal editors, and so on) and networking at socials.

❑ Schedule lunches and dinners with officers of professional organizations to discuss your research and any grant opportunities during conferences.

❑ After year 2, begin to volunteer and run for positions on national professional committees.

❑ Submit a proposal to serve as a guest editor for a major journal.

Learning to Say No

A lot of service, professional, and community service activities are available to faculty, especially nursing faculty. Female and ethnically diverse faculty are often asked to serve on university, national, and community committees to ensure representation of women and minorities. Although it feels good to be asked and is an honor, it is important to be selective, protect your professional and personal time, and not overextend your service commitments. Therefore, it is perfectly fine to say no or, "Thanks for asking, but I have made other commitments at this time. Please consider me in the future." Most individuals will understand that the timing is not good for you and that you need to protect your time. They also will appreciate that you are not agreeing to serve on the committee when you already are overextended. Agreeing to serve on a committee and then not attending or contributing will damage your professional reputation.

Chapter Checkup

❑ Do I have an understanding of the different types of required service (e.g., departmental, college, university, and professional)?

❑ Do I have a realistic understanding of the time commitment of the service requirements?

❑ Can I recognize when outside employment is affecting my professional and personal life?

❑ Have I prepared a sample short-term calendar (e.g., weekly) and a long-term calendar (e.g., semester, academic year) for a visual of service requirements?

❑ Do I have a clear understanding that I must be selective and not over-commit?

❑ Have I looked at how I can best utilize my time to get the most bang for my limited availability (e.g., getting double duty out of a conference attendance)?

❑ Can I identify my limits and know when to say no to requests to serve on committees?

TEACHING

ELEMENTS OF TEACHING

1. Faculty impart knowledge to students.

2. Faculty teach in different settings, including classrooms and online.

3. Faculty must establish and honor office hours.

4. Faculty must review student evaluations and adjust their teaching accordingly.

Chapter 2 introduced the importance of scholarly activities, including the importance of developing a line of research, writing for publication, presenting your work at professional conferences, and obtaining grant funding to support your research. Chapter 3 covered fulfilling the service requirements set forth by your institution. This chapter is dedicated to the scholarship of teaching.

The Value of Teaching

Merriam-Webster (n.d.) defines *teaching* as guiding the studies of students; imparting knowledge; instructing by precepting, example, or experience; and causing to know something. Teaching is an important part of tenure-line faculty members' role. Depending on the university, the area of teaching might be considered as important as the scholarly activities of writing, presenting, and obtaining grants, or it might be weighted as being either more or less important.

It is important to note that some universities stress the importance of teaching, research, and service by differentially weighting each area. By applying a different weight to each area, the university is essentially letting faculty and the public know what it values most. For example, some universities use a weighting scale or a percentage scale to determine the value of teaching, scholarship, and service during the tenure probationary period, merit, and post-tenure review. Specifically, if teaching is weighted or valued more compared to research and service, then teaching will receive a higher weight/value compared to service. Four-year and two-year universities are more likely to place a higher value on quality instruction and service compared to universities with a Carnegie Doctoral classification (2015), which place a higher value on research.

The following examples illustrate how universities weight teaching, research, and service differently.

Example 1: Susan (Four-Year Carnegie Baccalaureate Institution)

Susan is preparing for her first promotion and tenure (P&T) review and needs to submit evidence related to teaching, research, and service. As she is developing her P&T materials, she discovers that teaching receives a much higher weight compared to research and service. In fact, her university has indicated that teaching is weighted at 70%, service is weighted at 20%, and research is weighted at 10%.

The P&T committee has developed a rating scale to assess her teaching, research, and service, and it places more weight on teaching and requires a higher rating compared to research and service. Susan needs to spend the majority of her time focused on demonstrating the innovativeness and quality of her instruction and student learning outcomes. She just cannot just include course evaluations (even if they are excellent) in her P&T materials. Susan needs to demonstrate how her course lectures, assignments, and assessments are directly linked to student learning outcomes.

Because service is given higher value compared to research, Susan needs to demonstrate how her professional service contributes to the mission of the university. Ideally, she also should demonstrate how her service contributes to her instruction. For example, if she is working at a local hospital once a week in the critical-care unit, she should develop case studies that are based on real situations or demonstrate new medical techniques she has learned in her courses.

Example 2: James (Carnegie Doctoral Classification University)

James is completing his third year as an assistant professor at a major university. The university values teaching and research equally, while placing less value on service. He is required to develop a P&T notebook that includes three sections (teaching, research, and service).

James has known since the first year that the university P&T committees will rate each area using a Likert scale, from 1 (Poor) to 10 (Exceptional). He must receive a rating of 7 or higher in the areas of teaching and research and a rating of 5 or higher in the area of service. James needs to spend a significant amount of time demonstrating how his research informs his teaching and vice versa in his P&T notebook. For example, James's area of expertise is family-centered care; he has published several research articles on this topic as well as written a book chapter.

In his P&T materials, he should show how he has incorporated his research into his course. For example, James links his research with other published research on the topic during course lectures, his students write several annotated bibliographies based on research published on family-centered care, and he requires students to read his chapter as part of the course readings.

 Do you know the value placed on teaching at your institution compared to the value placed on research and service? You should explore this issue and make sure you clearly understand the expectations prior to your P&T review.

How Teaching Is Evaluated

Teaching is often evaluated by using students' course evaluations of faculty at the end of each term, peer-review evaluations of faculty, and administrative evaluations of faculty.

Here are examples of the peer and administrative questions that you will be reviewed on:

- Does the instructor develop and present content consistent with the objectives?

- Is the instructor knowledgeable and current on the course content?

- Is the instructor prepared for each class?

- Does the instructor present material in an organized manner?

- Does the instructor give explanations clearly, distinctly, and concisely?

- Does the instructor use different teaching methods?

- Does the instructor use different types of technology and/or teaching materials appropriately?

Often the evaluation ratings are on a Likert-type scale with predetermined questions. Regardless of how teaching is valued, it should be considered a very important aspect of your career. You have a great deal of knowledge and are becoming an expert in your area of professional practice, so it is important that you share your knowledge with others. The following are a few pointers regarding teaching and course evaluations as they relate to promotion and tenure:

- It is helpful to demonstrate how research and service enhance instruction and vice versa when developing P&T materials.

- Students will often send you cards and emails complimenting your teaching. Keep these in a notebook for future reference related to P&T and merit.

- It is important to be very clear in your P&T materials about how research and service enhance your teaching. After your P&T materials leave the department, it is likely that faculty representing other disciplines will be evaluating your teaching. So, it is important to clearly demonstrate how your research and service enhance your classroom teaching.

- Determine how course evaluations are interpreted in your department, college, and university. For example, some universities leave it up to the department to set the criteria for determining whether course ratings are poor, good, or exceptional. It also is important to know whether your course evaluations must be at or above the mean for your department, college, or university.

- Ratings are greatly influenced by the number of students enrolled in your course. Therefore, average course ratings can be greatly skewed by a single low rating. Say that one student completes a course evaluation and rates all 15 items on the evaluation much lower compared to other students. After review, the instructor finds that the student in the course gave her a 1 (Poor) on all items, whereas most of the other students in the course rated her as a 4 or 5 (Outstanding) on all items. First, it is possible that the student was confused and thought a 1 was actually an Outstanding rating. Second, it is not uncommon to have at least one or even two students rate much lower compared to other students, no matter how solid your instruction was. Finally, indicate clearly in your P&T document that the course had a small number of students. P&T committee members often will scan ratings looking for outliers, so provide an explanation for the lower course ratings for the specific course.

- Always read written comments on course evaluations. Even if the majority of student comments are positive, develop a plan for addressing any negative comments. Even if you only receive one or two negative comments, work to improve in future courses, with the goal of having all positive comments. Keep a record of how you respond (e.g., make changes to the course syllabus, revise a lecture, modify an exam, change your office schedule, etc.) to negative comments. By demonstrating that you are responsive to student feedback (positive and negative), you show P&T committees that you are strongly focused on student learning. Finally, be sure to indicate in your P&T materials how you responded to negative student comments.

Teaching Successfully in Different Settings

To be successful at teaching, you must devote time to perfecting it. Most faculty do not start out to be great teachers—although it would be wonderful if they did; instead, they perfect the art of teaching over time. It can be intimidating to stand in front of a class full of students. It can be even more frightening when you are teaching a difficult course or a course with tedious content. The good news is that most seasoned faculty have experienced difficult students, undesirable class times, and even some unwanted classes, and they will most likely be happy to share their experiences and give you some tips to avoid some of the same occurrences.

Although many people think it is most desirable to teach in the classroom face-to-face with students, education is changing. Classroom teaching is still predominate, but online teaching or hybrid teaching (a combination of online and classroom) is becoming more and more popular and desirable by faculty and students. Perhaps you have experienced both ways of learning during your own educational path and now have developed a preference. There are rewards and challenges with all types of teaching; just as students might prefer one style to another, faculty also differ in their preferences in teaching.

The National Center for Education Statistics (2014) reported that 5.4 million students took at least one online course in the fall of 2012. The data also showed that graduate students were more likely to study exclusively online versus undergraduate students.

Teaching in the classroom may be rewarding to faculty who enjoy face-to-face contact with students for specific periods of time each week. Generally, faculty develop lectures and handouts in preparation for class. Faculty teaching online courses also may need to prepare PowerPoints to supplement video lectures and/or readings. Depending on the course and level you are teaching, you might have anywhere from 10 to 200 students or more. Large groups of students may make it challenging for faculty to promote active engagement. On the other hand, small groups of students may not always provide enough diversity to promote good discussion. Teaching in the classroom requires you to be present for a specific time frame each week. One positive aspect of teaching in the classroom is that once your class is done for the day, you are generally free to work on other activities, attend meetings, or hold office hours.

SUGGESTIONS FOR TEACHING IN THE CLASSROOM

- Begin each class with a five-minute recap of the previous class. Allow for one or two questions. This allows everyone in the class to begin at the same place.

- End each class with a two- to three-minute recap of the lecture, and remind students of your office hours.

- Offer different types of teaching methods and assignments (e.g., lectures, case studies, group activities) to keep things exciting and to avoid student boredom.

- In addition to the traditional assignments (e.g., quizzes, exams, group projects, and papers), offer a variety of creative assignments (e.g., video or web development, creative writing essays, interviewing a client/patient, journaling, crossword terminology, role-playing, etc.).

- Consider holding one-hour, weekly study sessions for the entire class.

Teaching online is different than teaching in the classroom. For instance, you might have students living in different time zones and have expectations that you are available at all times (24/7). You also need to have all of your lecture material, exams, and so on loaded in the online course program. You need to determine whether students are permitted to work ahead of the assignment timeline. Also, instructors are often expected to read all discussion-board entries and then respond to each student or write out a group response. Online teaching requires good time management and patience. On a positive note, you can teach online from anywhere and at any time. From our personal experiences, teaching online tends to be more work than teaching in the classroom.

Whether teaching an on-campus or online course, allow to students to complete a two- to three-question mid-term evaluation of the course. Taking care of course concerns midway through the semester can eliminate frustrated students at the end of the semester. Anecdotally, taking care of any course issues midway through the semester can also improve overall course evaluations.

SUGGESTIONS FOR TEACHING ONLINE

Communication is key. Because faculty tend to have to type out their responses to students (which can take a great deal of time), consider these suggestions to avoid time-consuming duplicate responses:

- Add a frequently asked questions (FAQ) sheet to your announcement page. Refer students to that page when FAQ are asked via email, on a discussion board, or during an activity.

- Offer group chats or other online group discussions so students can meet with you to get their questions and concerns addressed in a single meeting. These online group meetings will save you hours of typing out individual responses and give students an opportunity to connect the faculty member's name with a face.

- Consider adding a video update twice a week to your online course. Faculty can record a video with assignment clarifications, updates, or answers to student inquiries and then upload the video to the online course.

- Rather than respond to each student individually, some faculty choose to include their answers to student inquiries and student discussion boards in one weekly written update. This update is then uploaded into an announcement at the start or end of each week.

- The syllabus is the contract with the student, so communicate what your availability will be. If you do not plan to respond to students on the weekend, state so in the syllabus. Indicate to students that they need to plan their work accordingly.

Hybrid courses are a combination of both classroom and online teaching. Some faculty believe it is the best of both teaching methods, because the instructor is not required to be in the classroom each week, and it allows instructors to teach from remote locations.

All teaching delivery methods have positive and negative aspects to them. You might not always have the option of choosing which teaching delivery method you end up doing, so you will want to be prepared and knowledgeable about all methods.

Prepping for Your Classes

The American Faculty Association (2012) indicates that faculty should expect to spend two to four hours of prep time for every hour of class instruction. However, Wankat and Oreovicz (2000) believe you can prepare too much. Their recommendation for lecture prep time is two hours for a new lecture and 30 minutes for established lectures. Wankat and Oreovicz provide an interesting insight to lecture preparation, which is to start early to prevent a panic mode and to devote a specific amount of time to the crucial points of the lecture. It takes time to become proficient at teaching.

Don't be afraid to ask for help or even shadow a more experienced faculty member to gain better insight into the teaching process. Most universities have a specific department that can help you design courses, better your teaching, and ultimately improve student course outcomes.

At some point in your teaching career, you will be asked questions that you may not know how to answer, or you may simply not know the response. Admit when you do not know something, and assure students you will research the answer and respond to them in a timely manner.

The following are a few other pointers to assist with course preparation:

- Incorporate real-life examples in your courses to facilitate understanding and interest.

- Avoiding lecturing during every class session. To maintain interest, vary the course activities from week to week.

- Don't interpret a lack of response or engagement by students during lectures as their being unprepared or uninterested. Students may be struggling to grasp concepts or just might be tired from studying for a major exam in another course.

- Evaluate each lecture or course session to determine whether there are ways you can improve and increase student learning.

- Some lectures or course sessions will just be busts. It might be better to scratch them and start over by preparing a different lecture on the topic.

- If you have a teaching assistant (TA), use him or her! Don't be afraid to assign the TA sections of a lecture to teach or use the TA to assist in developing lectures.

- Don't overuse a teaching method (e.g., group discussions, games, guest speakers, etc.) that created high interest with students. If overused, students will lose interest fast and realize that you may be using the method to avoid prepping for the course.

Establishing Office Hours

You need to set aside time for office or consultation hours, allowing opportunities to meet with students enrolled in your courses and to provide specific student-faculty interaction. Some departments require faculty to have at least 8 hours of office time per week. This is something you need to inquire about and then establish which day or days work best for you. You might be able to accomplish other tasks (e.g., class preparation, answering emails, scheduling meetings, etc.) during this time, but it generally is a time specifically to meet with students. Although it might be nice to engage in casual conversation with students during office hours, this particular time should be kept more formal and tend to the tasks of helping students be better prepared for class, reviewing exam results, counseling students who are not progressing well, and providing encouragement.

Weimer (2015) finds that students do not always make use of scheduled faculty office hours. Results of a study indicated that students either did or did not utilize office hours based on one of the following reasons:

- Faculty did not provide feedback during office hours.

- The hours and location were inconvenient.

- The course was listed as a 100 or 400 level.

- The class size was small.

- The class was required for a declared major.

- Additional or alternative office hours were offered.

- Students could alternatively contact the faculty using email.

- The course was traditional or blended.

- The faculty was perceived to be approachable or unapproachable.

- Information had been clearly or not clearly explained in class (Griffin et al., 2014; Weimer, 2015).

The points Griffin et al. (2014) provide are worthy of consideration for all faculty when establishing office hours and developing teaching styles. Consider that you may also meet with students in small groups to discuss a topic or issue that pertains to all of them. If your office does not accommodate small groups of students, consider reserving a classroom or meeting space. Keep in mind that the availability of technology, blackboards, or whiteboards may be limited, so plan accordingly.

SETTING OFFICE HOURS

- Set office hours. (Note: Be available two different times throughout the week.)

- Post your office hours in the syllabus, on your office door, and in the course itself (e.g., as an announcement).

- Post office hours at the beginning of the semester and throughout the semester.

- Make it clear to students whether office hours are drop-in or whether they need to make an appointment.

HOLDING AN EFFECTIVE OFFICE VISIT

- Prior to the visit, communicate how much time you are willing to give to each student. For example, if your office hours indicate one-hour availability, then it makes sense that each student should be given a limited amount of time to accommodate multiple students. So, in this example, offer each student 10 minutes.

- Communicate with students that they need to come prepared. Students should have their questions written out (sending them to you prior to the office meeting is even better).

- Set a good example. If a student schedules a visit, you should be punctual and begin the meeting on time.

- Ask the student how many questions he or she has. If the student has one or two easy questions, then go through each one. If the student has more complicated questions, prioritize them. Address as many as you can in the time period, and then schedule another time to meet.

- Have a blackboard or whiteboard available to illustrate examples to the student.

- Have the course textbook available to guide the student to specific readings or examples.

- At the end of the meeting, physically hand the student something. This simple gesture says, "You are important to me, and I am giving this information to you." For example, offer your business card for future contact, a previously developed "how to study for my class" tip sheet, or a worked-out example of the problem.

- Script a closing statement. This might sound funny, but practicing how to end a student meeting is important and can keep you on schedule. You want to be available to as many students as possible, but you don't want the student to feel rushed. One example is, "That is all the time that we have today. Have I provided clarification to your questions?"

- If the student needs more time, schedule another meeting before he or she leaves.

- Prior to ending the session, give positive praise. Students are often intimidated by faculty and avoid reaching out, so it is important to make a student feel at ease. For example, state, "Thanks for stopping by to get your questions answered. I am impressed that you took the initiative."

Dealing With Sensitive Issues

If you are meeting to discipline a student or to discuss a sensitive subject, always have another person present at the meeting. This is for your protection as well as the student's. You may also want to keep the office door open when appropriate for safety reasons and set an established time limit for the meeting. If the meeting needs to be confidential, meet in a conference room instead of your office. Other students and faculty will often stop by or wait outside your office door if they know you are meeting with a student. If a difficult situation escalates to the point that the student is out of control, it may be best to stop the meeting and reschedule for another time.

The following are some additional pointers for meeting with difficult students or disciplining students:

- If you are going to have another faculty member meet with you and the student, be sure to let the student know this before the meeting.

- Have copies of policies and procedures or university links on your computer readily available so you can review them with the student. Make sure you have reviewed university policies and procedures before meeting with the student.

- If you are meeting with a student via FaceTime, Skype, or phone, it is important to ask whether anyone else is present on the other end before starting the meeting. Also, it is important to be aware that students can record most electronic video sessions.

- Always follow up on what was discussed with a short email, and indicate at the end of the meeting that you will be sending the student a short email summarizing the meeting.

Clinical or Practicum Requirements

Some faculty are teaching courses that have clinicals or practicum requirements in addition to in-class and online instruction. Faculty who have courses with clinicals or practicum components need to balance their time to meet their other commitments of teaching, scholarly writing, and service. You might need to make adjustments to time dedicated to writing and research to accommodate the supervision requirements of clinicals. However, being assigned to clinicals may also provide opportunities for research.

Clinicals are courses that a student must complete to meet two different, yet related, requirements. Clinical courses have a didactic (e.g., lecture) component and a clinical requirement (e.g., 90 in-hospital hours). Faculty assigned these types of courses have to balance the additional stress and time commitment of traveling to and from the clinical site. In addition to the the time spent at the clinical site, time will be spent on clinical preparation and student clinical assignments.

Graduate-level courses have practicum requirements. Students complete practicum hours, a type of capstone for graduate students, in order to meet the requirements of the specific department and of the graduate school. These practicum hours are completed at a specific site, depending on the degree. Sites could include a university, acute-care hospitals, physician clinics, or even community-based facilities. Nursing practicum hours are generally limited to one semester, but the number of hours can range widely. For example, in certain nursing concentrations (e.g., leadership or education), practicum hours may be as few as 180 for the semester. Yet for a Nurse Practitioner (NP) degree, the practicum hours could be 600 to 900. Faculty must adjust their schedules to accommodate the added supervision for practicum courses.

 Clinical and practicum courses are not isolated to nursing. Psychology, education, engineering, etc., all have such requirements. Consider the added responsibility when making your calendar and planning your schedule.

RESEARCH IDEAS AT CLINICAL SITES

- Interprofessional networking at clinical sites is important.

- Identify clinical needs that could be further researched.

- Identify gaps in research when investigating clinical issues.

- Communicate your interests to colleagues at the clinical sites, and reach out to others who share similar interests.

- Learn the clinical sites' Internal Review Board (IRB) process.

Making the Most of Student Evaluations

If you teach, students will likely complete evaluations of your teaching and lectures. Each university has a requirement for student evaluations of faculty, including the type and number of questions asked. The evaluations are anonymous. Faculty generally receive a copy of the evaluations at the end of each term. The intent of evaluations is to provide feedback to faculty for course improvement and or faculty teaching style. However, students are not always nice when providing feedback and may also include personal attacks on the faculty. Take heart: Many faculty experience this, and although negative comments are hurtful, you will survive.

See Chapter 11 for more information about how to deal constructively with negative student evaluations.

You might be inclined to not read the evaluations, but you really should read them with an open mind. If there is constructive feedback provided that you can carefully consider for making changes, then do so. We can all do some things better. Keep in mind, though, that some things are out of your control. If you are reading the same types of criticism year after year, then you really may need to make changes in your course or teaching style. You might also want to seek help from more experienced faculty to improve your teaching and/or course.

Faculty pursuing the tenure process are generally required to obtain at least an average rating on all teaching evaluations throughout the probationary period. Not everyone agrees with using student evaluations of faculty as part of the tenure process. Flaherty (2016) believes that student evaluations of faculty are unreliable, show biases, and create a culture of grade inflation to obtain higher evaluation scores.

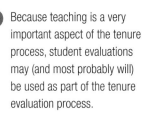

Because teaching is a very important aspect of the tenure process, student evaluations may (and most probably will) be used as part of the tenure evaluation process.

Regardless of how faculty feel about being evaluated by students, it is a long-standing practice that will probably not go away any time soon. Consider that you will not be able to please all students all the time, nor should you. Your job is to teach them what you know and prepare them for the workplace. Students might not realize how much they were taught or how valuable the teaching was until they have graduated and are using what they have learned. Your focus should be on simply doing the best you can at the time you are doing it, seeking help when needed, and continually making updates and changes that improve your overall teaching and the experience for the students.

SUGGESTIONS ON HOW TO ENHANCE TEACHING

- Review course evaluations to identify strengths and weaknesses (each semester), looking for consistent themes.

- Review student-written comments for specific themes, and develop a plan to address them in future courses.

- Request a senior faculty (who has an excellent history in teaching) to observe your course and provide informal recommendations.

- Observe other instructors (known to have excellent teaching evaluations), and schedule other classroom observations.

- Have two or three other faculty review your course syllabi, course assignments, exams, and course instruction and provide informal feedback.

- Conduct an informal anonymous course evaluation at mid-term that includes open-ended questions.

- Be sure to provide timely and constructive feedback on all assignments, even if you utilize grading rubrics.

- Email students at least one or two times per week to provide reminders of upcoming assignments, including helpful tips, and to indicate accessibility (e.g., available by email, Skype, phone).

- Reach out to students who are struggling in your course, and provide opportunities for them to work with you.

- Consider adding a study session outside the class's instructional time.

- Take advantage of any university training to improve your instruction.

- Have a strong understanding of university policy related to plagiarism and academic dishonesty.

- Have a strong understanding of university support services (e.g., writing lab, student disability services, supports for culturally and linguistically diverse (CLD) individuals, etc.).

- Consider incorporating a variety of assignments that meet the needs of different types of learners in your course (e.g., quizzes, developing presentations, speeches, case studies, and so on).

- Include fun activities within the course to facilitate learning and offer students the ability to be creative (e.g., puzzles, group projects).

Chapter Checkup

❑ Do I have an understanding of how teaching is weighted at my university?

❑ Do I understand the different ways to approach teaching in the classroom versus online?

❑ Have I established office hours?

❑ Have I considered the time commitment of clinicals or practicum courses and adjusted my schedule accordingly?

❑ Do I understand the importance of student evaluations?

❑ Do I have a full understanding of how to adjust my teaching based on my student evaluations?

❑ Do I have a clear understanding of how to prepare for class?

References

American Faculty Association. (2012). Hours for teaching and preparation rule of thumb: 2-4 hours of prep for 1 hour of class. Retrieved from http://americanfacultyassociation.blogspot.com/2012/02/hours-for-teaching-and-preparation-rule.html

Carnegie Classifications of Institutions of Higher Education. (2015). Carnegie classification descriptions. Retrieved from http://carnegieclassifications.iu.edu/classification_descriptions/basic.php

Flaherty, C. (2016). Bias against female instructors. *Inside Higher Ed.* Retrieved from https://www.insidehighered.com/news/2016/01/11/new-analysis-offers-more-evidence-against-student-evaluations-teaching

Griffin, W., Cohen, S., Berndtson, R., Burson, K., Camper, M., Chen, Y., & Smith, M. A. (2014). Starting the conversation: An exploratory study of factors that influence student office hour use. *College Teaching 62*(3), 94–99. doi:10.1080/875675555.2014.896777

Merriam-Webster. (n.d.). Full definition of teach. Retrieved from http://www.merriam-webster.com/dictionary/teach

National Center for Education Statistics. (2014). Enrollment in distance education courses, by state, fall 2012. Retrieved from http://nces.ed.gov/pubsearch/pubsinfo.asp?pubid=2014023

Wankat, P., & Oreovicz, F. (2000). How much is enough? Too much class preparation may not pay off. *ASEE Prism Teaching Toolbox, 10*(1), 41. Retrieved from http://cgi.stanford.edu/~dept-ctl/tomprof/posting.php?ID=257

Weimer, M. (2015). Why students don't attend office hours. *Faculty Focus.* Retrieved from http://www.facultyfocus.com/articles/teaching-professor-blog/students-dont-attend-office-hours/

5

DEVELOPING A LINE OF RESEARCH

ELEMENTS OF DEVELOPING A LINE OF RESEARCH

1. Ensures degree (PhD, EdD, DNP) consideration.

2. Decision on a broad or narrow line of research.

3. Positive external letters are required for promotion.

4. External reviewers can be difficult to obtain.

5. DNP programs are less likely to prepare researchers.

Faculty applying for promotion from associate to full professor are expected to demonstrate a line of research, whereas most assistant professors are just beginning to define their line of research. A faculty member's *line of research* is considered a series of highly focused studies on a specific topic or problem. A line of research can be very narrow or broad. In some institutions, faculty can also have more than one line of research; more than two or three lines, though, are not as common.

> *"A faculty member's line of research is considered a series of highly focused studies on a specific topic or problem. A line of research can be very narrow or broad."*

> *"In some institutions, faculty can also have more than one line of research; more than two or three lines, though, are not as common."*

For example, a faculty member's line of research could focus on studying the effects of a specific vaccine on infant growth or be more broadly defined as research focused on studying the diets of adults with Type II diabetes. Or, a faculty member may have one line of research focused on the treatment of autism and a second line of research focused on the use of simulations to enhance learning among undergraduate nursing students. Although many faculty change lines of research throughout their careers, some faculty maintain the same line of research throughout their entire careers. For example, a beginning faculty member may change her line of research after conducting several studies because there is limited publication potential in her topic area or the research is unlikely to result in external funding. An associate or full professor may decide to change a line of research because the current line of research is no longer of interest. In short, faculty lines of research often change.

"A beginning faculty member may change her line of research after conducting several studies because there is limited publication potential in her topic area or because the research is unlikely to result in external funding."

More prestigious universities sometimes hire faculty who have very specific lines of research, which were often started while they were completing their dissertation and doctoral degree. More often than not, though, first- and second-year faculty are just beginning to establish a line of research, and it is very difficult to establish a line of research on five or six publications. Therefore, many institutions do not expect faculty being considered for promotion from assistant to associate to have a fully established line of research.

The following are a few additional comments related to establishing a line of research:

- It is difficult to demonstrate a line of research if you are not the senior author on a majority of your publications. It would be hard to make the case that a line of research is *yours* if you are not the senior author of several of your publications.

- It is helpful to define your line(s) of research and indicate how each publication is consistent with your line(s) of research to external reviewers. Typically, universities require faculty to select several of their publications that best represent the quality and rigor of their research, which will be sent to external reviewers. In addition, faculty usually include a narrative describing their research to the external reviewer.

External Review Letters

At institutions where *external letters* are considered an essential part of the promotion and tenure (P&T) process, established lines of research are important. Specifically, external letters are typically requested from experts in the field who have lines of research similar to the faculty being reviewed for promotion or promotion and tenure.

The university depends on the external reviews as a way to gain an independent, unbiased review of faculty research. Institutions commonly request reviewers to address the following issues when conducting external reviews:

- Does the faculty member's research make significant contributions to the field of nursing? If so, how?

- Discuss the rigor and specific contributions of the published research to the field of nursing by the faculty member.

- Is the research being conducted sustainable as a line of research?

- Given the faculty member's line of research and quality of publications, is it likely that he or she will receive external funding if promoted?

- Are the quality and level of scholarly productivity equivalent to the faculty at your institution who have been promoted from associate to full professor?

- Would you recommend that the faculty member be promoted to full professor? Why or why not?

Having a clearly defined and established line of research is essential to receiving good external letters. It also important for faculty, especially at universities with a Carnegie Doctoral classification, to publish in high-impact journals. In terms of external funding, faculty who have lines of research consistent with an external funding agency or foundation's mission are more likely to receive funding. The following are some important considerations related to external letters:

- Typically, universities with a Carnegie Doctoral classification are more likely to require external letters during the promotion process. However, it is becoming more common for universities with Carnegie Master's and Baccalaureate classifications to request letters.

- Some universities require external letters as part of the P&T process from assistant to associate professor.

- External reviewers are sometimes asked to review teaching and service efforts too, not just research.

- It will be difficult to receive positive external letters if you are not the senior author on a majority of your publications. Specifically, it would be difficult for external reviewers to indicate that your publications have a significant impact on the profession or that you are capable of independent research if you do not have several senior-authored publications.

- Universities usually have very specific procedures and criteria as to how external reviewers are selected and what materials need to be submitted for review. For example, a university may require the department chair or P&T committee to identify and select external reviewers. Or, the faculty member may be able to submit a list of names of possible reviewers, and the department chair and P&T committee select external reviewers from the list. At other institutions, the external reviewers are selected from separate lists generated by the faculty member and the department chair or P&T committee. There can also be a combination of both, meaning that the faculty member selects a few external reviewers and the department chair selects a few different external reviewers.

- External reviewers are typically anonymous to the faculty member. Although faculty may submit a list of potential external reviewers, in the end, they do not know which reviewers agreed to complete an external review. When a faculty member is allowed to read an external letter, all identifying information is typically blacked out.

- It can be difficult to find faculty at other institutions to serve as external reviewers, especially if the faculty member being reviewed will eventually know who conducted the external review. In fact, institutions will inform potential reviewers at the time of a request whether the external review will remain anonymous or whether the faculty member will know who conducted the review. Not surprisingly, it may take several lists and a significant amount of time to find external reviewers. Typically, universities require at least two to three external reviews.

The Doctorate of Nursing Practice Project

There are an increasing number of registered nurses returning to college and earning doctoral degrees, including a doctorate of nursing practice (DNP) degree (AACN, 2012a). Unlike the PhD (independent original research) and EdD (research focus in education), the intent of the DNP is to prepare nurse "experts in population-based practice," which is practice that's focused on a specific group of people, to advance the education of nurses to the practice doctorate (AACN, 2004, p. 9). Most programs focus on advanced clinical practice, healthcare policy, and education (Grey, 2013). Nurses with DNP degrees now number more than 1,600 (Dennison, Payne, & Farrell, 2012). Today, DNP nurses are holding positions in administration, education, and beyond. However, Grey (2013) questions whether the original intent of the DNP educational role is really being achieved, because so many DNP graduates are employed in positions not related to population-based practice.

The educational process for DNP students differs from that of PhD and EdD students in that the DNP student may complete a final DNP practice application-oriented final project rather than an Internal Review Board (IRB)–approved dissertation (Kirkpatrick & Weaver, 2013). A larger concern might be the lack of consistency in the expectations and quality of the DNP education and projects, which might lead to concerns for success if the graduate is seeking a tenure-track position in a school of nursing (Melnyk, 2013; Udlis & Mancuso, 2015).

According to the American Association of Colleges of Nursing (AACN, 2006), the DNP student completes a practice application-oriented final DNP project, which prepares the graduate for a practice-focused position. The AACN (2015) also expects DNP students to complete a minimum of 1,000 hours of postbaccalaureate practice hours as a component of their program. Melnyk (2013) believes the DNP project should focus on leadership projects, evidence-based projects for change, and evidence synthesis. There is also some controversy concerning whether DNP graduates should hold tenure-track or clinical-track positions (AACN, 2012b).

You must consider the university in which you plan to practice when factoring whether, as a DNP nurse, you should seek a tenure-track or alternatively a clinical-track position. In research universities, tenure is generally awarded based on the research contributions the faculty make during the probationary period. Because DNP programs are relatively new, it is still to be determined whether DNP-prepared faculty have the knowledge and skills to conduct rigorous original research and achieve tenure. However, in universities where teaching is the priority and may lead to tenure, DNP-prepared faculty may be more successful in achieving tenure (Grey, 2013).

It would be incumbent upon students seeking doctoral degrees and subsequently tenured faculty positions to make careful decisions when seeking doctoral degree education so their future plans for employment can be fulfilled. Only you know how you work and how determined you are to succeed. Sometimes a strong determination and the willingness to work hard is half the battle.

Chapter Checkup

❏ Do I have an understanding of the difference between the PhD, EdD, and DNP?

❏ Do I have an idea of what my line of research will likely be?

❏ Do I understand the nature and purpose of external letters?

❏ If my degree is a DNP, do I have the research background and skills to accept a tenure-track position that focuses on research?

References

American Association of Colleges of Nursing (AACN). (2004). AACN position statement on the practice doctorate in nursing. Retrieved from http://www.aacn.nche. edu/publications/position/DNPpositionstatement.pdf

American Association of Colleges of Nursing (AACN). (2006). The essentials of doctoral education for advanced nursing practice. Retrieved from http://www. aacn.nche.edu/publications/position/DNPEssentials.pdf

American Association of Colleges of Nursing (AACN). (2012a). Fact sheet: The doctor of nursing practice (DNP). Retrieved from http://www.aacn.nche.edu/ media-relations/fact-sheets/DNPFactSheet.pdf

American Association of Colleges of Nursing (AACN). (2012b). Doctor of nursing practice (DNP) programs: Frequently asked questions. Retrieved from http:// www.aacn.nche.edu/dnp/faqs

American Association of Colleges of Nursing (AACN). (2015). The doctor of nursing practice: Current issues and clarifying recommendations. Retrieved from http:// www.aacn.nche.edu/aacn-publications/white-papers/DNP-Implementation-TF-Report-8-15.pdf

Dennison, R. D., Payne, C., & Farrell, K. (2012). The doctorate in nursing practice: Moving advanced practice nursing even closer to excellence. *Nursing Clinics of North America, 47*, 225–240. doi:10.1016/j.cnur.2012.04.001

Grey, M. (2013). The doctor of nursing practice: Defining the next steps. *Journal of Nursing Education, 52*(8), 462–465.

Kirkpatrick, J. M., & Weaver, T. (2013). The doctor of nursing practice capstone project: Consensus or confusion? *Journal of Nursing Education, 52*(8), 435–441.

Melnyk, B. (2013). Distinguishing the preparation and roles of the Doctor of Philosophy and Doctor of Nursing Practice graduates: National implications for academic curricula and health care systems. *Journal of Nursing Education, 52*(8), 442–448. doi: 10.1016/j.outlook.2010.11.001

Udlis, K. A., & Mancuso, J. M. (2015). Perceptions of the role of the Doctor of Nursing Practice-prepared nurse: Clarity or confusion. *Journal of Professional Nurses, 31*(4), 274–283. doi:10.1016/j.profnurs.2015.01.004

6

WORK/LIFE BALANCE

ELEMENTS OF WORK/LIFE BALANCE

1. Balance work and personal responsibilities.

2. Protecting personal time during breaks is essential.

3. Summers can be quite demanding.

4. Responsibilities increase as faculty progress toward tenure and promotion.

5. Submission of manuscripts can be time-consuming.

In the previous chapter, we discussed developing a line of research; the differences between a PhD, EdD, and DNP; and the DNP project. In this chapter, we address the importance of a work/life balance. With the high levels of nurse burnout (Buerhaus, Donelan, Ulrich, Desroches, & Dittus, 2007) being attributed to demanding workloads and inadequate social support (Duquette, Kerowc, Sandhu, & Beaudet, 1994), it makes sense to consider the requirements of academic positions (e.g., teaching, research, service, and grant writing). Therefore, the importance of meeting professional responsibilities while maintaining a personal life cannot be overstated. Developing a good work/life balance will be essential as you progress through the six- or seven-year probationary period when in a tenure-line position.

Research has shown individuals who maintain a balance between their work and personal life are more likely to be more productive employees (Lazar, Osoian, & Ratiu, 2010). This same logic can be applied to individuals working in higher education. Maintaining an appropriate balance between work and home can lead to success in your academic career. Because the tenure-line process is generally a seven-year period, it is good to develop work habits that will result in quality publications, grants, teaching opportunities, etc., while allowing you to focus on your family and personal life when you're away from the university.

Burning out is different than rusting out. When someone is burning out, that person is experiencing too much stress related to daily routines, tasks, or courses, whereas someone who is rusting out no longer finds the daily routines, task, or courses interesting.

CHECKLIST!

- ❏ Plan your time.
- ❏ Work ahead when possible.
- ❏ Secure a faculty mentor.
- ❏ Secure family support.
- ❏ Take time for some fun.
- ❏ Get proper rest.
- ❏ Eat a good diet.

Consider these helpful tips to achieve that work/life balance:

- Always keep your Outlook calendar up-to-date. It is much easier to have colleagues "invite" to you to meetings electronically than to play phone tag (which can be stress-inducing).

- If possible, have due dates/times at 5:00 p.m. (this will eliminate answering questions after-hours, which is an infringement of your personal time).

- Avoid having assignments due on Sunday evenings, because students will contact you over the weekend. Again, this will eliminate answering questions during your personal time.

- Keep two calendars at all times. The first calendar is your workweek and includes detailed meetings, teachings, and scholarly activities. This calendar also has your personal time marked, meaning, if the work day ends for you at 7:00 p.m., then from 7:00 p.m., the calendar is marked as "personal." No more work after 7:00 p.m. The second calendar includes your academic calendar, which includes semester or quarterly start dates, any breaks (i.e., national holidays, and fall or spring breaks), and semester end dates (e.g., fall, spring, and summer). Having a fully completed annual calendar will provide you, at a glance, with the entire academic calendar.

Look at your calendar when you are submitting manuscripts. Many manuscripts require revisions, which may fall during your personal breaks or time off. To avoid revisions during a break, submit the manuscript immediately before the break (during the break, the reviewers will be reviewing the manuscript), or submit the manuscript when you return from your break.

Managing the Academic Year

A university's or college's academic year usually includes the fall and spring semesters, unless the institution uses a quarter system. Generally speaking, most faculty are quite busy during the academic year with their teaching and service requirements, so they often conduct their research, write manuscripts, and complete presentations during the summer months. During the academic year, your assignment may vary, but generally faculty are expected to teach several courses and serve on department, college/university, and or professional organization committees in addition to pursuing their scholarly work. Typically, faculty have the option of teaching during the summer or taking their summers off from teaching and service. Interestingly, due to the large number of students admitted to nursing programs, it seems that nursing faculty are often pressured to teach during the summer. The following are a few pointers regarding summer teaching:

- Summer teaching tends to be quite time-consuming, even if faculty agree to teach only one course. It is important to remember that summer courses are more instructionally compact. The same amount of material is typically covered in a 5- or 10-week course during the summer as during the same 16-week course taught during the academic semester.

- Undergraduate students who enroll in summer courses tend to represent bimodal groups, with one group representing students who have to retake courses and the other group representing students who are highly motivated and want to get ahead on their coursework. Having two distinct groups in a summer course can make a summer course more demanding to teach.

- At many institutions, the amount that faculty are paid for teaching a summer course is not worth the time away from family. It is important to determine whether the break from the demands of teaching is worth more than the stipend. Specifically, will taking a break help you avoid burning out or rusting out? If so, it's time well spent.

- Summer is a good time to catch up on writing. Many faculty find they are more likely to write for extended periods during the summer compared to the academic year. Also, many faculty write and submit one to three manuscripts during the summer and then complete the rewrites and resubmissions, if needed, during the academic year.

As you progress through the tenure-line probationary years, it is not uncommon to experience increased expectations related to teaching and service. You may also want to teach during the summer or may be required to teach during the summer term. Many universities take it easy on beginning assistant professors during their first year in higher education. For example, they may limit the number of committees, assign them three sections of the same course to limit preps, or even reduce the number of courses they teach each semester. However, tenure-track faculty should expect to be assigned more responsibility as the years toward tenure continue. In other words, year 1 of the tenure-line process will have far less responsibility than year 7.

TENURE-LINE YEAR 1

❏ Establish teaching methods.

❏ Develop course lectures.

❏ Establish a line of research.

❏ Complete or update Collaborative Institutional Training Initiative (CITI) training for the Internal Review Board (IRB) process.

❏ Research possible grant-funding sources.

❏ Seek publication and presentation opportunities.

TENURE-LINE YEAR 2

❏ Continue to refine teaching methods.

❏ Continue to revise and improve course lectures.

❏ Write one IRB proposal in your established line of research.

❏ Submit an abstract for a presentation.

❏ After IRB approval, complete the research study.

❏ Submit for a small internal grant (e.g., seed money).

❏ After the research study is complete, write up the results.

❏ Submit manuscript for publication.

TENURE-LINE YEAR 3

❏ Continue as above, and write a second IRB proposal or continue with the first IRB.

❏ Conduct research study, and write up the results.

❏ Submit manuscript for publication.

Making Time for Research

As we have discussed, many tenure-line and tenured faculty conduct their research in the summer, write manuscripts, and conduct presentations at various professional conferences. But the summer may also be a time to rejuvenate. Conducting research in the summer must be well thought out. You must take into consideration the type of research you are doing, where you are obtaining the population, and whether they are available during the summer months.

For example, if you are investigating the school nurse role, the summer months may not be the ideal time to initiate a study, because school nurses may not work during the summer months. There are many great organizations that conduct wonderful conferences where you may present your research results, or you may also earn continuing education credits. You will need to plan and select conferences, carefully because conference fees and additional costs may range from hundreds to thousands of dollars. Although some universities refund faculty for presenting at conferences, some universities do not refund faculty, so these expenses may be out of pocket. You will also need to know what your university and tenure committee consider "meeting" requirements when considering attending or presenting at a conference. Some committees require that faculty present at national and or international conferences and do not place as much value on local or state conferences, so it is important to know the expectations you will be required to meet.

You may or may not be teaching in the summer, or, if you do, you may not be teaching a full load. Regardless, you will need to balance your time well if you are going to be effective in conducting some of your research during this time period. It is important to establish what you realistically plan to accomplish over the two- to three-month summer period and then devise a plan to achieve your goals. It is easy to have grandiose ideas related to the amount of writing you plan to accomplish over the summer but they may not be realistic. Once you have established a plan, stick to it as much as possible. Set aside time each day to work on your research but avoid trying to accomplish too much at one time. Many tenure-line faculty attempt to do too much and become overwhelmed which may lead to feelings of failure or worse dropping off tenure. For example, it would probably not be wise to try and conduct a research study that requires traveling a long distance multiple times to collect data because you will have limited time in the summer months.

> *"It is important to establish what you realistically plan to accomplish over the two-to three-month summer period and then devise a plan to achieve your goals."*

ESTABLISHING A REALISTIC PLAN (IN A TWO- TO THREE-MONTH PERIOD)

- Plan to focus on one study at a time.

- Get IRB approval well in advance, because some IRBs do not meet during the summer months, or as often.

- Develop a timeline of when every item is due.

- Develop a Gantt chart, which is a horizontal chart that tracks the progress of projects and workload.

- Print informed consent forms and any other required forms well in advance.

- Secure participants well in advance.

Manuscript Writing/Grant Writing/Rewrites

After collecting and analyzing your data, you need to write the results and submit manuscripts for possible publication. Do not expect to sit down and write a manuscript in a couple of hours. Writing manuscripts takes a significant amount of time, even for the most accomplished authors. It is not uncommon to spend 40 to 60 hours or more to write a 25- to 30-page manuscript.

It can be helpful to follow a routine when writing. For example, establish a place to write that is free from distractions. This may be in your home or office. You may need to turn your phone off and tell others you will be writing and should not be disturbed. It takes time to get into a writing mind-set, and if you're interrupted, it will take you additional time to get back into the writing mode. Do not be surprised if you experience difficulty getting started, which is often called "writer's block." However, you might start by developing an outline or by putting some initial thoughts on paper to help the process along. Pretty soon you will have the basis to start writing a paragraph, and then a page, and so on.

You should expect to write and rewrite your manuscripts several times. It also is recommended that you have a trusted colleague read and edit your manuscripts prior to your submitting them to professional journals. Please be courteous to the individual reading and editing your manuscripts, and give him or her at least one week to complete editing a manuscript. It is very frustrating to be asked to review a manuscript with a short turn-around time. Also, do not debate edits or suggestions with the individual who read and edited your manuscript.

Typically, someone who reads and edits a manuscript for a colleague does the following:

- Asks the author exactly what he wants in terms of reading and editing the manuscript. For example, when I am asked to read or edit a manuscript, I ask the author whether he wants me to provide general comments or to perform a hard edit. I also ask whether he wants me to correct grammar or focus on major areas (e.g., mention gaps in the literature that are not covered in the manuscript, point out methodological problems that need to be addressed, or provide suggestions on the interpretation of statistics) that need to be addressed.

- Asks the author which journal she plans to submit the manuscript to. If the individual does not know, I ask whether she wants journal suggestions.

- Asks when the author wants the suggestions and edits. If it is fewer than two weeks, I politely request that he ask someone else to read the manuscript.

- If I return a manuscript and provide significant input and the author starts to argue or debate comments I have made, I politely say, "Take or ignore my suggestions, it is up to you." However, it will be the last time I take my time to review and edit a manuscript for the individual.

If you are grammar challenged or writing in a nonnative language, it might be best to hire someone to proof and correct the spelling and grammar for you. There are people on university campuses who moonlight and edit manuscripts for a nominal fee. This may be well worth your time and money. Also, some universities offer free APA or MLA formatting prior to submission. In addition, some national organizations offer writing retreats, such as the National League for Nursing (NLN, 2016) and the Midwest Writers Workshop (Midwest Writers Workshop, 2016).

NEED HELP WITH WRITING?

Try these sources:

- ❏ National League for Nursing's Scholarly Writing Retreat

- ❏ Midwest Writers Workshop (www.midwestwriters.org)

- ❏ Your institution's writing center

- ❏ Work with a colleague who is an accomplished writer

Once you are ready to submit a manuscript, it is extremely important that you select the journal that best fits your topic. Be sure to read and follow the manuscript-submission requirements prior to uploading the document. If the journal requirements state that the manuscript must be within 1,200 words, then do not submit a 2,000-word manuscript, as it will most likely be rejected without review.

Submitting a manuscript can take several hours. Most journals now require manuscripts to be submitted electronically. The process of submitting a manuscript requires more than uploading your file. You need the contact information of all the authors; you need to respond to several questions related to ethics; and you may need to upload your manuscript in sections (e.g., abstract, tables, figures, etc.) instead of as one complete document. Some journals require all authors to sign in and respond to several questions about their involvement in the preparation of the manuscript and ethical questions.

Make sure you understand the peer-review process and how long it typically takes for a journal to make an editorial decision. Once you have officially submitted the manuscript, you may add the information to your vita (CV) as *submitted* without listing the journal. When you receive your peer-reviewed manuscript, read the reviewer comments carefully, and make the necessary suggested changes if you plan to resubmit the manuscript. You may not always agree with the reviewer comments and do not have to make the changes suggested. But keep in mind that if you do not make the suggested changes, you most likely will need to submit the manuscript to a different journal. Only you can decide whether you want to make the suggested changes and resubmit the manuscript. In most cases, the suggested changes are made to strengthen the manuscript and help authors improve their writing.

If a manuscript is rejected, consider the reviewer comments, make changes if desired, and submit the manuscript to another journal. Do

Some journals will make an editorial decision within three to four weeks, while other journals take three to six months or more. Unless you have time to wait on a three- to six-month editorial decision, do not submit to these journals.

You can only submit the manuscript for review to one journal at a time. So it's important that you select a journal that best fits your topic and the quality of your study.

not take the rejection decision personally; sometimes the article is simply not a good fit for the selected journal. If you receive an acceptance letter, then rejoice! You may still need to make some minor corrections to the manuscript prior to final acceptance and publication. The journal will send a final proof of the manuscript, requiring you to go through the manuscript and answer any queries (questions). The journal will provide an estimated date for publication. You should retain a copy of the email or letter, enabling you to track your manuscript. After the manuscript has been accepted for publication, it now can be listed as *in press* on your CV. Your manuscript may be printed in either a hard-copy or online journal format, depending on the journal. Once the manuscript is in print or published online, it is considered *published*.

You may want to retain copies of your acceptance letters and published articles for your personal records, because some university tenure committees require that hard copies of the documents be placed in a binder during the annual promotion and tenure (P&T) review. You need to be aware that sometimes the publication process may take one to two years from the time you submit to when you have a published article; therefore, it is very important that you are continually working on manuscripts and research.

Writing grants and securing external funding are often requirements at institutions with a Carnegie Doctoral classification. In
fact, at some universities, faculty are required to acquire external
funding to support their line of research. Identifying potential
grants and reading requests for proposals (RFPs) can be an arduous and time-consuming process. If you have never written
a grant proposal, then it would be a good idea for you to attend
some grant-writing workshops. Universities generally offer grant-
writing workshops for free, or you can attend a workshop course at
a professional conference or pay for a grant-writing course with a
nonprofit or for-profit organization.

You might also obtain some help through your university's contracts and grants office. Once you have identified the need for
grant money and possible grant sources, the next step will be to
write the actual grant proposal. Some organizations have specific
deadlines for grant-proposal submissions, certain organizations
send out RFPs, and others offer open-ended submission dates.
You will need to follow the grant-submission guidelines carefully.
Typically, grant proposals include a narrative, goals and objectives,
outcomes, assessment, biographical info, and budget sections.

Normally, the grant proposal will then be submitted through the
university's grant and contracts office for review and submission
to the granting organization. You will need to keep a record of
the grant proposal, submission dates, and assigned grant numbers
for your records. You may also be asked to make changes to your
grant proposal and or adjust your budget. Again, you may need to
print these documents and add them to your tenure-line review
binder or online reporting system. If you are awarded grant monies, the award may come directly to you or to the grant office at
your university. If you receive the monies, you will need to submit
the monies to your institution's grant office. As you use the monies, you will submit the receipts to the grant office for payment or

reimbursement. Money that is not used should be returned to the granting organization. Most grant-offering organizations require that you submit a final report detailing how the money was used and outlining the outcomes of your research.

In summary, books have been written on how to write grants. Also, the topics discussed here should be considered a very general overview of the grant process. The following list provides a few comments related to grants, promotion, and tenure:

- Pursue internal grants within your institution prior to applying for major external grants. Internal grants are much easier to attain, and many institutions provide specific feedback, allowing faculty to resubmit during the next grant cycle.

- Internal grants can often lead to larger external grants. Many granting agencies are looking for some prior success with grant-funded research.

- Look for opportunities to be written into major grants being submitted by senior faculty who have a history of successful external funding.

- If your university does not require external funding for promotion and tenure, it is likely in your best interest to focus on publishing in referred journals.

- Always visit with your department chair when you are deciding to write a grant proposal and pursue external funding. Department chairs will give you good advice on whether it is in your best interest to spend your time writing and pursuing major grants prior to being tenured and promoted.

It may seem odd to include manuscript writing, grant writing, and rewrites in a chapter covering work/life balance, but what we are trying to stress here (no pun intended) is that you need to consider every aspect of these requirements when working through each. For example, when you are watching television in the evening with your family, this is not the time to "quickly" submit a manuscript (see the comment about submissions).

Institutional Review Board

The IRB is in every university/college, and all researchers must submit their research-study proposals to the IRB for review. Often research is considered exempt, but if not, you will need to follow the established protocol carefully. Initially, you will need to complete the CITI training according to the rules established by your institution. Once you have completed the training, you will receive a certificate of completion. You must retain this certificate as proof of completion. When submitting a research-study proposal, you will need to follow the institution's IRB submission protocol. Once the IRB committee has reviewed your proposal, you will receive notification of study status and an IRB proposal number. You will need to retain this information for your records. If you make any revisions to your proposal or study documents, you will need to submit a change document (i.e., amendment) and again wait for approval prior to continuing your research.

When you have completed the study and do not plan to continue with future work for the study, you will be required to complete and submit a final report to the institution's IRB committee, which closes your study. A notification that the study was closed should follow, and this document should also be retained for your records. If you think you may want to continue in the future with a specific study, you may have to renew your IRB approval (typically on a yearly basis).

A couple of final comments regarding the IRB:

- Developing and submitting an IRB proposal is time-consuming, and many researchers are surprised by the detail required by the IRB when submitting a proposal. It literally can take as much time to submit an IRB proposal as it does to write a manuscript!

- Expect to rewrite an IRB proposal several times, especially if the research involves minors.

- Expect to respond to questions from the IRB, especially if the study is fairly sophisticated. It is important to note that the IRB is often composed of faculty who represent different disciplines. Therefore, they may not understand the scope and nature of your proposed research.

- Avoid taking comments from the IRB personally. The role of the IRB is to protect research participants, the university, and you. However, at times, the IRB can be fairly direct with its comments and feedback when corresponding with researchers.

We often hear first-year tenure-line faculty make unrealistic comments about IRB proposal development, such as, "I know the IRB deadline is coming up, so I will work on that proposal while my daughter is taking a nap," or, "I can quickly put that together this weekend." But the reality is you simply cannot do an adequate job with distractions or quickly pull together an IRB proposal. Working on an IRB proposal takes focus. To help you achieve work/life balance, the next sections include some suggestions.

Balancing Personal, Family, and Year-Round Commitments

As we addressed in the first chapter, if you are granted a tenure-line position, there will be expectations during the seven-year probationary period that will affect your personal and family life. It is better to understand these commitments so you can make an informed decision and determine whether a tenure-line position is right for you. There will always be tenure-related commitments and personal, family, and other outside obligations that pull you in many different directions. There may be things you would like to do, and then there is the reality of what you are able to do with regard to the tenure requirements and your personal life. There has to be work/life balance, and it is very easy to allow things to get out of balance when pursuing promotion and tenure.

OBLIGATIONS

Personal	Work
Spouse	Teaching
Children	Publication
Church	Presentations
Outside activities	Grants
	Service

At many universities, the tenure expectations include demonstrating that you are able to conduct original research, publish, obtain grant funding to support your research, and present at national and international conferences. Depending on your institution's tenure requirements, some of these categories may be weighted more heavily than others. You will need to pay close attention to what your tenure review committee deems most important and concentrate on excelling in those areas. You will most likely need to make some sacrifices during this process. You may not be able to take a long vacation or attend every sporting event for your children. You may need to spend evenings and weekends, holidays, and summers working. However, rest times are equally as important. A realistic meaningful discussion with your family is very important so that everyone understands that some sacrifices will need to be made by everyone if you are to be successful.

We do stress that you take time out for yourself and your family to relax and regroup. It is easy to become consumed with working, and that promotes some very unhealthy habits. Giving up everything that is important to you can result in resentment and frustration for you and your family.

Chapter Checkup

☐ Do I have an appreciation for work/life balance?

☐ Have I completed an assessment of my own work/life balance issues?

☐ Do I have a complete understanding of the time commitments involved in manuscript and grant writing (including the required rewrites)?

☐ Do I have a plan for those work/life issues that may need some assistance, including childcare?

☐ Do I understand what goes into managing an academic year?

References

Buerhaus, P., Donelan, K., Ulrich, B., Desroches, C., & Dittus, R. (2007). Trends in the experiences of hospital-employed registered nurses: Results from three national surveys. *Nursing Economics, 25*(2), 69–79.

Duquette, A., Kerowc, S., Sandhu, B., & Beaudet, L. (1994). Factors related to nursing burnout: A review of empirical knowledge. *Issues in Mental Health Nursing, 15*(4), 337–358.

Lazar, J., Osoian, C., & Ratiu, P. (2010). The role of work-life balance practices in order to improve organizational performance. *European Research Studies, 13*(1), 201–214.

Midwest Writers Workshop. (2016). Retrieved from http://www.midwestwriters.org/faculty/

National League for Nursing (NLN). (2016). National league for nursing: Scholarly writing retreat. Retrieved from http://www.nln.org/centers-for-nursing-education/chamberlain/scholarly-writing-retreat

PROMOTION AND TENURE DECISIONS

ELEMENTS OF PROMOTION AND TENURE DECISIONS

1. Universities review faculty differently during the probationary period.

2. There tends to be an administrative line of review and a faculty line of review.

3. A variety of decisions and recommendations are made by committees and administrators.

4. Views are changing regarding pursuing early promotion and tenure.

5. Termination can lead to different employment situations.

Faculty are usually reviewed each year during the probation-ary period. The level of review varies greatly from university to university. At some universities, the review process can be quite extensive—faculty might have to prepare materials and submit them electronically or as a hard-copy notebook. The materials are then typically reviewed at all levels (e.g., department, college, and university) within the university system. At other universities, the materials may just be reviewed by the departmental promotion and tenure (P&T) committee, and the letters are sent up to be reviewed by the dean, provost, and president.

The Promotion and Tenure Review Process

Not all universities review faculty on a yearly basis. For example, some universities might review faculty progress toward tenure on a two- or three-year cycle during the probationary period. Still other universities might review faculty on a yearly basis only at the departmental level, and then on certain years (e.g., years 3 and/or 5) during the probationary period also review faculty at the college level. At the end of the probationary period (typically year 6 or 7), faculty are usually reviewed at all levels within the university system, starting at the department level and going all the way to the president.

Make sure you understand the promotion and tenure review process at your institution, including how often it occurs and what's expected. Don't be afraid to ask questions if the policies are not clear. These are good questions for your department chair, chair of the P&T committee, or professional mentor.

Typically, faculty are reviewed by P&T committees composed of peers within the university and by administrators. Therefore, there is typically what is called an administrative line of review and a faculty line of review. Department chairs might not participate in the deliberations of the department P&T committee; if they do participate, it is typically in an *ex officio* capacity. A similar process may be followed at the college level, where the dean participates in the college P&T committee deliberations as an *ex officio* member. The department chair and the P&T committee may be required to work together to write a decision letter, but it is more common for department chairs and departmental committees to write separate decision letters.

At most universities, departmental and college committees—as well as chairs and deans—write letters recommending a specific action (e.g., satisfactory progress, tenure, promotion, termination, and so on) that are reviewed by university committees and upper administration. Typically, the provost or president makes the final decision regarding the recommended decisions. At some institutions, however, the provost or president makes the final recommendation to the board of trustees, who approve the promotion and tenure decision. Figure 7.1 illustrates a common decision-making process for a faculty member at the end of her seven-year probationary period at a major university.

Based on Figure 7.1, it is easy to see that the promotion and tenure process takes time. It is not uncommon for faculty not to know the final decision related to promotion and tenure until May or June of the year after they submitted their promotion and tenure material (submitted in October or November the year before). It also illustrates why faculty often feel anxious until they receive the final decision letter. Essentially, because there are so many levels where decisions are made, faculty often worry that they will receive a negative decision.

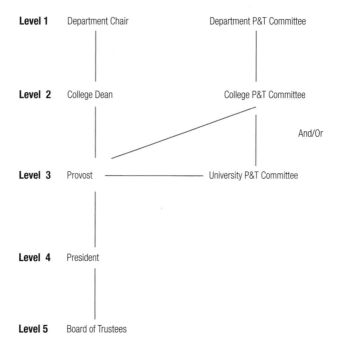

Figure 7.1. Typical faculty tenure-line decision-making process.

Common Recommendations/Decisions

There are many decisions and recommendations that committees and administrators can make. Faculty should review university promotion and tenure documents to understand each possible decision and the meaning of the decisions. Faculty at the majority of institutions should also be aware that a recommendation made by an administrator or committee at a lower level might not be the same as a recommendation at a higher level within the system. In other words, administrators and committees at higher levels do not simply rubber-stamp lower-level decisions. This section covers some of the most common recommendations/decisions that exist.

Satisfactory Progress Toward Tenure

During the yearly tenure review, the most common recommendation is "satisfactory progress toward tenure." (It is important to note that universities have different terms for faculty making satisfactory progress toward tenure.) A "satisfactory progress toward tenure" recommendation at the department level does not necessarily guarantee that the same recommendation will be made at the college or university level. However, it is rare for a satisfactory progress recommendation made at the department level to be reversed at an upper level.

Faculty receiving a positive letter should read the letter closely. It is very common to receive a positive letter that reviews a candidate's strengths but also includes recommendations for areas for improvement. If there are areas in need of improvement, the faculty must address them prior to the next annual review or prior to the end of the probationary tenure review decision. The letter serves as documentation of the committee's or administrator's recommendations for areas of improvement. Faculty who ignore the recommendations are not likely to fare well during the next yearly tenure review or during the end-of-probation tenure decision.

Unsatisfactory Progress Toward Tenure

Universities have different approaches and procedures for informing faculty that they are not making satisfactory progress toward tenure. An "unsatisfactory progress toward tenure" decision essentially means that faculty demonstrate a lack of progress in teaching, research, or service. It is important to note that a lack of progress toward tenure decision can be based on a lack of progress in all the aforementioned areas or a lack of progress in only one area. For example, an assistant professor who demonstrates excellence in research but consistently receives low course evaluations might be given an "unsatisfactory progress toward tenure" decision. Faculty also might receive a positive decision one year and the next year receive an unsatisfactory decision. For example, a faculty member who publishes three manuscripts in year 2 and then has no publications during years 3 and 4 is likely to receive an unsatisfactory letter from the department P&T committee during the fourth-year review.

Many faculty become quite frantic and discouraged after receiving an "unsatisfactory progress toward tenure" decision. Such a decision can have different meanings and consequences, depending on the institution. For many institutions, the letter is essentially a warning—a wake-up call, so to speak—to notify the faculty member that he or she needs to address areas of weakness or deficiency (e.g., needs to increase scholarly productivity). In those cases, the faculty member often needs to address the deficient areas or demonstrate an increase in scholarly productivity by the next tenure review or by the end-of-probation promotion and tenure decision. In the majority of cases, faculty respond to and meet the required areas of improvement. However, improvement often requires an immense amount of time commitment and work. For example, if the faculty member is behind in number of publications, he or she must catch up while also meeting the next year's required number of publications. Once you've fallen behind, especially in terms of publications, it takes an extensive amount of work to catch up!

> *"An 'unsatisfactory progress toward tenure' decision is essentially a warning—a wake-up call, so to speak—to notify the faculty member that he or she needs to address areas of weakness or deficiency."*

Fortunately, most institutions require committees and administrators to provide clear feedback related to areas in need of improvement to help the candidates. Also, the majority of administrators and P&T committees want to see junior faculty be successful.

Therefore, although they make objective decisions regarding promotion and tenure and rely on the promotion and tenure documents to drive the decisions, the majority of administrators and committee members are empathetic on how negative decisions affect junior faculty. Outside the promotion and tenure process, it is not uncommon for administrators and faculty to offer assistance and mentoring to help faculty meet promotion and tenure requirements.

Again, it is important to review department, college, and university documents related to an "unsatisfactory progress toward tenure" decision to understand exactly what it means at your institution. At one institution it could be a warning letter, at another it could be a loss of a year toward tenure, or at a third it might lead to termination if more than one "unsatisfactory progress toward tenure" decision is made during the probationary period.

Termination or Denied Promotion With Tenure

Although recommendations for termination are uncommon during the six- or seven-year probationary period, they do occur. In fact, recommendations for termination can occur during the first-year tenure review, when the faculty member has only been at the institution for a short period of time. Again, this is fairly rare! When administrators or department committees recommend termination, there typically are extenuating circumstances. The following are some common reasons for termination or denial of promotion and tenure:

- The department determines that the line of research a faculty member is pursuing is inconsistent with the line of research the faculty member was hired to conduct.

- The instructor consistently receives very poor course evaluations and has not responded to remediation, mentoring, or training to improve instruction.

- There is a complete lack of or a low level of scholarly productivity.

- There is a major ethical violation (e.g., faking research data, plagiarism, ghost grading of assignments, and so on).

- There is a lack of participation/attendance in departmental meetings or committees.

- The faculty member consistently misses or cancels courses.

- The faculty member does not respond to student emails, consistently is late grading assignments, or exhibits a lack of rigor when teaching online courses.

- The faculty member minimally meets requirements but does not excel in teaching, research, and service.

Faculty who receive a decision for termination often are not surprised. Typically, there have been signs of the impending decision. For example, prior unsatisfactory progress toward tenure decisions, multiple meetings with the department chair, development and implementation of remediation and accountability plans, and several attempts at mentoring the candidate, of which all or some have not been successful, usually result in a termination decision.

Many faculty are devastated by a termination decision, which is quite understandable. However, termination can result in self-reflection related to working in higher education or in a change of employment that better matches the faculty's career goals.

Although leaving an academic position can be highly stressful professionally and personally, faculty tend to find an another academic position that better matches their strengths. For example, the faculty member who struggles at conducting research but is an excellent instructor would be better suited to finding employment at an institution that has a primary mission of teaching. The positive perspective on termination is that things tend to happen for a reason, and the majority of faculty tend to be much happier, professionally and personally, after making a career change, whether they made the decision or it was required due to a termination decision.

It also is important to note that most universities allow faculty to stay an extra year after a termination decision. Specifically, the faculty member is notified that his or her position will be terminated within a year, starting at the end of the spring semester. For example, a faculty member is notified in December that the department P&T committee's decision is termination, and the president affirms the decision the following April. That candidate will typically have until the end of the following spring semester to find new employment. Most university faculty senates and unions have negotiated the additional year after a termination decision to protect faculty and to avoid unforeseen hardship on the faculty member. The following are a few additional comments related to termination:

- Not all universities allow faculty to stay an additional year after a termination decision. It is important to review the faculty handbook and promotion and tenure guidelines before accepting a position.

- Some universities will allow faculty to stay an additional year, but their status at the university will change. For example, policies might dictate that the faculty member will no longer continue within a tenure-track position but will be switched to a full-time contract position.

- Faculty load might change. Instead of being given load for research, the faculty may be given four courses to teach each semester. Many universities take the perspective that if a faculty member is terminated for low scholarly productivity, it does not make sense to give him or her load for research the following year.

- Faculty may also see service eliminated the following year, which also makes sense. If a faculty member will be leaving at the end of the next academic year, it does not make sense for him or her to chair or participate in committees. It also would be fairly awkward to have a faculty member who has been terminated serving on committees within the university.

- Don't expect a merit or salary increase. Universities will typically not allow merit or salary increases for faculty who are staying the additional year after a termination decision.

- A faculty member's salary may actually decrease. It is not uncommon for some institutions to convert a faculty member's salary so that it is consistent with the salary of of full-time contract faculty member.

- Some universities will allow faculty to come off the tenure-track line and work as a full-time contract faculty member indefinitely.

Early Promotion and Tenure

Historically, it was unheard of for faculty to seek early promotion and tenure. The risk was just too great! Specifically, the majority of institutions would allow faculty to apply for early tenure and promotion but with penalty—it would lead to termination if they were not granted early tenure and promotion. However, now more universities are including language within promotion and tenure documents that allows faculty to apply for early promotion and tenure without penalty. Faculty may apply but are not terminated if denied early promotion and tenure. Typically, the university that allows early tenure and promotion without penalty will not consider early tenure requests until after the fourth year.

Faculty are often allowed to apply for early promotion and tenure only once during the probationary period. This primarily is due to the large rate of attrition that occurs among assistant professors during the first six to seven years of employment. Universities have found that assistant professors are more likely to make a career move during the first six or seven years, even if they are making good progress with tenure. For example, faculty often change academic positions early because of a lack of spousal employment opportunities, a desire to increase income, or a dislike of the local community (e.g., limited shopping, limited healthcare, lack of a cultural support group, and so on).

Institutions are realizing that faculty attrition is expensive. Therefore, as an incentive to retain high-caliber faculty, many institutions are increasingly encouraging early promotion and tenure. This approach makes a lot of sense. If a faculty member is an exemplary instructor, is publishing and presenting at a high rate, and has excellent service, why wouldn't a department, college, and university want to retain that person?

The decision to apply for early promotion and tenure should be made in consultation with the department chair and/or the chair of the department P&T committee. These individuals can give some indication of how the credentials of a faculty member compare to other faculty who have pursued and been granted early promotion and tenure. It would be very difficult to attain early promotion and tenure without the support of the department chair.

Appealing Negative Promotion and Tenure Decisions

Every university has its own internal process related to appeals and reconsiderations. Faculty need to know the process, the steps within the process, and the timeline. The following are some additional comments related to appeals:

- Appeals are very complicated and require an extensive amount of time and preparation on the part of the faculty member and the university.

- Although appeals are complicated and require an extensive amount of time, faculty who have had a negative promotion and tenure decision often feel compelled to utilize the appeal process, especially if the negative decision comes at the end of the probationary period.

- It is usually the faculty who has to demonstrate that treatment was unfair, that promotion and tenure policies and procedures were not followed, or that discrimination occurred. Proving you were treated unfairly is very difficult to do, whereas documenting that a committee did not follow the promotion and tenure policies and procedures can be easier. Claiming discrimination also can be very difficult and can result in the university's human resources, compliance, or legal department's becoming involved in the appeals process.

- The success of appeals varies greatly from one institution to another. Based on our experiences, it is difficult to win an appeal, especially based on claims of unfair treatment. It is important to remember that universities have been working on and fine-tuning their promotion and tenure policies and procedures for decades. They also have had attorneys to review and approve their documents for years. Most promotion and tenure policies and procedures are immune to legal challenges.

- Many faculty will ask whether they should seek an attorney. This is a very difficult question to answer. Some universities restrict individuals from outside the university from participating in the appeal process. However, other universities might allow it. Still, it is common for universities to require faculty to follow the internal processes and procedures. Therefore, we are not recommending that you retain an attorney or not retain an attorney. Every situation tends to be unique and requires an independent decision on the part of the faculty member.

Chapter Checkup

❑ Do I have an understanding of the different promotion and tenure decisions that are made at my university?

❑ Do I know whether my university allows faculty to apply for early promotion and tenure?

❑ Do I understand the appeal policies and procedures at my university?

❑ Do I understand the termination process at my university?

PROMOTION AND TENURE DECISIONS WHEN CHANGING INSTITUTIONS

ELEMENTS OF PROMOTION AND TENURE DECISIONS WHEN CHANGING INSTITUTIONS

1. Considerations must be made when applying to other institutions.

2. Faculty leave positions for a variety of reasons.

3. Politics affect decisions when applying and leaving.

4. Effective negotiation is important.

5. Decisions can have long-term consequences.

It is fairly common for faculty, especially assistant professors, to change institutions prior to being granted promotion and tenure. Faculty leave one institution to pursue employment at another institution for a variety of reasons. Here are some of the more common reasons for changing institutions:

- No spousal accommodations

- Increase in pay at a new institution

- Lack of institutional supports

- Lack of fit with current institution

- Difficulties with meeting promotion and tenure requirements

- No openings at institutions of primary interest when looking for positions

- Determination that higher education is not consistent with career goals

- Little to no interest in conducting research

- Lengthy commute

- Family stressors (e.g., work time commitment too great)

- Health issues with family members (e.g., parents need assistance)

- Geographic location of institution

- Lack of cultural or religious groups within community

- Limited childcare

The Politics of Searching for and Accepting Another Position

Deciding to apply for an academic position at other institutions can become politically sensitive very quickly. Therefore, it is important to consider the politics of the current department and how they might affect your current position, any pending promotion and tenure decisions, and interaction with colleagues. The following points are helpful to consider before applying to other academic positions:

- Whom can you use as a professional reference at your current institution? Depending on the reasons you are applying for positions, you might not be able to utilize references at your current institution. For example, if you are struggling with research at your current institution, received a negative promotion and tenure decision, or have poor collegial interactions, it is likely you will need to look outside your current institution for professional references. Former instructors, colleagues at other institutions, and individuals you have worked with in clinical settings can serve as professional references.

- Search committees are quick to recognize when applicants do not use professional references from their current institutions. Therefore, if you don't, be prepared to address why during the interview. Someone on the search committee is going to ask why you do not have any professional references from your current institution. It is important to be honest when answering the question.

- It is very difficult to keep job searches confidential, especially if you use individuals at your current university as professional references. In our experience, it is almost impossible to conduct a job search without others finding out at some point. Therefore, just assume that at some point, someone will find out, even if you asked the individuals who are writing reference letters to remain confidential. Politically, it is important to decide when to let your department chair, colleagues, and program chair know you are applying for other positions. Depending on your situation, it might be best to inform your department chair before applying for other academic positions, or it might be best to inform your department chair after you have agreed to an interview. In other cases, it might be best to wait until you have a job offer that you are seriously considering.

- Department chairs hate surprises. In our experience, most department chairs, although they are disappointed a faculty member is searching for another position, are supportive. However, be prepared to assure the department chair he or she is not the reason you are seeking employment at another institution. Most department chairs want to maintain a positive collegial and professional relationship, even if you take a position at another university. Also, it is important to remember that you are just informing the department chair that you are applying for other positions; he or she knows that applying and an accepting a job offer are two different conversations.

- It is important not to play games or "cry wolf." We have worked with faculty who tend to apply for jobs every year since they have started, only to interview and turn down offers each year. Often, they get a job offer and are looking to use it to negotiate a higher salary or a different teaching load. In our experience, applying, interviewing, and receiving a job offer to gain an increase in salary is a risky game to play. It will typically work once and *only* once. If you are denied the salary increase and you are not serious about accepting the other position, you risk walking away with a bruised ego! Also, it is not fair to the institution where you interviewed. The other institution may lose the position, lose other prospective candidates, and feel used if you interviewed only with the goal of pursuing a salary increase at your current institution. Lastly, the nursing field is fairly small, and it will not take long for other institutions to learn that you have a history of applying and interviewing without accepting offers of employment.

- Don't assume that you will be invited for an interview or offered a position when you apply somewhere. Although there are a large number of posted academic positions in nursing each year, it is important to understand that search committees consider several variables when conducting job searches. For example, salary, area of specialization that needs to filled within the program, research potential, and more are taken into consideration.

- The grass is not always greener on the other side of the fence! We have found that it is sometimes good for faculty to apply and interview at other institutions. Faculty often find that their current position, department, college, and university are actually more supportive and have more resources compared to other universities where they interview. Specifically, assistant professors may not know how good they have it in their current position until they interview and visit other universities.

Department chairs and faculty have different reactions once you accept a position at another institution. These reactions might be shared with you directly, or you might hear about them indirectly. Although chairs and faculty are supportive most of the time, it is not uncommon to receive very different reactions to the news that you are leaving. Be prepared for the different reactions. Here are few of the more common reactions:

- *Anger*—Department chairs and faculty might respond with anger due to a feeling of betrayal. For example, it is not uncommon for chairs to feel that they invested a large amount of time and money in you, yet now you are leaving.

> Although experts differ on the exact cost of employee turnover, they do agree that the overall cost is high, ranging anywhere from 50% to 75% of the individual's yearly salary.

- *Bartering*—Department chairs might want to meet with you to find out whether they can barter with you to reconsider. For example, you might be asked what salary it would take to keep you or whether decreasing your teaching load over the next couple of years would convince you to stay.

- *Disbelief*—Faculty you work with closely might be in disbelief that you are actually considering leaving the university. They might ask, "How can you even think about leaving us; aren't we a great department?"

- *Shaming*—Some faculty might confront you and attempt to make you feel guilty about your decision. For example, someone might say, "Don't you feel bad about leaving us after all the work we did to help you publish?"

Negotiating a New Tenure and Promotion Agreement

Whatever the reason you decide to apply for and seek employment at another institution, you need to make several major decisions related to promotion and tenure. In fact, you need to be prepared to negotiate with the prospective institution prior to accepting a position so that you're placed in the best position to gain promotion and tenure. The decision to leave a current position, interview while continuing to teach and conduct research, continue to address family responsibilities, leave colleagues you have developed close working relationships with at your current institution, and negotiate with another institution typically results in a highly stressful period. However, it is important to stay focused on making good decisions regarding promotion and tenure with your prospective employer. It is important to consider the following issues during the negotiation and decision process:

- Does the institution allow faculty to transfer years earned toward tenure and promotion when coming from another institution?

- How important is it to you to bring years toward tenure and promotion as you transition to the new institution?

- Is it in your best interest to negotiate years toward tenure and promotion based on the expectations at the new university?

- If you decide to negotiate years toward tenure and promotion, how many years should you try to bring with you?

These are four fairly complex questions that are typically unique to each individual. Let's discuss the first question. It is common for universities to allow assistant professors as well as associate and full professors to transfer years toward tenure and promotion. However, the number of years can vary greatly from university to university. A couple of scenarios help demonstrate and highlight the complexity and uniqueness of each situation.

Scenario I: Disappointed

A second-year assistant professor in nursing has decided she wants to move closer to her aging parents and has applied to several universities within four hours of her parents' home. She has interviewed for and been offered a position at a fairly prestigious university. She has published only one article in the past two years and has no presentations. The primary mission of her current university is teaching. During her negotiations with the chair of nursing at the prestigious university, the chair is recommending that she not request years toward tenure or promotion to allow her additional time to pursue her scholarship related to research. The new department expects one to two refereed publications per year (on average) prior to recommending tenure and promotion to associate during the seventh year. The assistant professor is disappointed with this recommendation and dislikes the idea of losing two years of work within higher education.

Scenario II: Overly Qualified

A fourth-year assistant professor at a prestigious university has decided to apply for positions near her fiancé (an accountant) in another state. She has interviewed at a four-year private college with a very strong nursing program where the focus is on teaching. She has been publishing an average of two manuscripts per year and has several national presentations. She also serves on a couple of nursing journal editorial boards. The department chair at the private college has recommended that she request five years toward tenure and that she come in at the associate level with the goal of going up for tenure during her seventh year.

The two assistant professors have very different situations and need to make different decisions related to tenure and promotion with their respective employers. The disappointed professor needs to make a decision regarding whether her career goals are consistent with those of the prestigious university, where there is a strong focus on research and refereed publications. If she enjoys teaching and has little interest in conducting research, she should reevaluate her decision to accept the position at the prestigious university, although she would be able to move closer to her parents. It would be better to continue to apply to openings at other universities that emphasize teaching. However, if she decides to accept the position, she should respect the chair's advice and not bring any years toward tenure and promotion to her new position. This will allow her the most time to develop and implement research projects that will ultimately lead to journal publications.

The overqualified assistant professor also needs to make a decision related to whether the four-year college is consistent with her career goals. If she enjoys research and publishing, she needs to decide whether she will be happy at an institution that primarily focuses on teaching. Again, if she wants to conduct research, she needs to keep searching for other academic positions. If she decides to accept the position, then she will need to consider the chair's advice. Although the offer to come in as an associate professor with five years toward tenure is reasonable, she might want to reconsider. It is rare for a university to grant tenure prior to a candidate's starting a position, even if the candidate has an excellent record of teaching, research, and service.

Granting individual tenure at time of hire is more common with senior faculty positions and administration. The overqualified professor might want to reconsider the offer to come in at the associate level but accept the five years toward tenure. Why would anyone turn down an offer to be granted associate when they are currently at the assistant level? The answer is simple: money! Most colleges and universities include a substantial increase in salary when an assistant professor is granted promotion to associate. If the professor negotiates a nice salary that includes five years toward tenure with the rank of associate, she will not gain a substantial increase in salary until she is promoted to the rank of full professor. It would be better financially to come in at the assistant level and then apply for associate in two years when she goes up for tenure. Look at it this way: The $4,000 increase in salary when she is promoted to associate over 20 years (estimating a 2% increase per year) is worth a little more than $80,000! Given the assistant professor's level of productivity, it is highly unlikely that she would not be tenured and promoted during her seventh year. Therefore, not getting caught up in the title of being an associate professor in the short term pays off financially in the long term.

Scenario III: Not Much Difference

In this situation, a fifth-year assistant professor in nursing decides he wants to move closer to his children, who live in another state, so he can take advantage of visitation on the weekends. He currently is at a prestigious university and has applied to another prestigious university with similar publication, teaching, and service requirements. The chair has offered him the position at the assistant level with four years toward tenure. The chair also has offered him $5,000 more in salary than he is currently being paid for the academic year. The university aligns tenure and promotion and has a fifth-year review as part of the seven-year probationary period. The college and department promotion and tenure documents clearly indicate that publications, presentations, and grants at prior institutions will be considered as part of the fifth-year review and seventh-year promotion and tenure decision. The assistant professor has consistently published one manuscript per year, has one national presentation each year, and has written a small grant ($50,000), which was funded. When the assistant professor compares the two universities, there is not much of a difference in the promotion and tenure requirements. They also have very similar teaching, research, and service requirements.

This decision seems fairly straightforward: Accept the position, maintain the same level of scholarly productivity, and enjoy the

$5,000 increase in salary. However, it is not as straightforward as it sounds, and the assistant professor could be setting himself up for problems with promotion and tenure.

The issue is the fifth-year review. Most faculty are required to submit their materials for review by the department, college, and university promotion and tenure (P&T) committee each fall—typically sometime in October or November. In this scenario, the professor was granted four years toward tenure and will be starting his fifth year. Essentially, his fifth-year review will be from the time of hire until his materials are due in October or November, which is a very short time to publish, present at a national conference, or write a grant. Also, it is unlikely that the professor will have any student evaluations based on courses taught until after the fall semester. It places the department, college, and university (P&T) committees in a very difficult position. Essentially, the committees will be evaluating the professor on his scholarly productivity, teaching, and service when he worked at the other institution, which is most likely what they did at the time he was hired!

It also is important to note that the college and departmental documents indicated that prior scholarship would be *considered*. It did not indicate that prior publications would be *counted* toward promotion and tenure decisions. Therefore, there is no guarantee that the college and department committees will accept the prior publications. In fact, the committees could indicate that the professor must publish six to seven manuscripts by the seventh-year review to be granted tenure and promotion to associate! The assistant professor would do better to negotiate three years toward tenure and *require* in writing that the college and department (P&T) committees count prior scholarly activity, teaching, and service when making decisions related to tenure and promotion.

Making Your Decision

These three scenarios illustrate the complexity of promotion and tenure negotiations when changing from one academic position to another. It is important to consult with senior faculty, review promotion and tenure documents closely, and take time when making decisions related to promotion and tenure. Every decision tends to be highly individualized. In the end, you have to make the decision that is best for you and live with that decision.

Chapter Checkup

- Do I understand the underlying politics related to searching for a job at my institution?

- Am I prepared for the reactions once faculty learn that I have accepted a position at another university?

- Am I prepared to make a good decision related to promotion and tenure with my new employer?

- Do I understand the promotion and tenure policies at my new institution prior to accepting a position?

- Am I prepared to request that all agreed-upon negotiations related to promotion and tenure be in writing before accepting a position?

KEEPING TRACK OF SCHOLARLY ACTIVITIES

ELEMENTS OF KEEPING TRACK OF SCHOLARLY ACTIVITIES

1. Ensures that *curriculum vitae* (CV) is current

2. Ensures that tenure documents are easily accessible

3. Provides a mechanism for keeping organized

4. Ensures that published manuscripts and documents are organized

In Chapters 7 and 8, we discuss what happens if you need to drop off tenure line, are denied tenure, or need to move to another institution. In this chapter, we discuss the importance of tenure documents and how to maintain and organize your tenure documents as you move through the probationary period. Your tenure documents will consist of a compilation of the previous year's work and all your work since starting at your institution, which includes published manuscripts, grants, teaching evaluations, etc. The promotion and tenure (P&T) committee may also require a verification email/letter/notification of any manuscript or grant submitted, so it is a good idea to save copies of these types of notifications and communications.

> You will be required to submit your tenure documents to the department's P&T committee. The tenure documents are a compilation of your previous year's work and typically include all your work since starting at your institution. To avoid undue stress, staying organized throughout the year is a must and helps decrease your stress during the P&T review process. Depending on your institution's submission due date, you may have only a few weeks after the start of a new academic year to turn in these documents.

It is very important that you be well organized and diligent in maintaining your scholarly documents. Your institution will most likely have specific requirements for maintaining the documents electronically (e.g., an online submission program, flash drive, Dropbox, etc.) or in binders to hold the documents. You will also create and maintain a CV to record your accomplishments over your career. Regardless of the manner in which you compile the documents, it is necessary to be organized and meticulous in saving and organizing the documents.

Keep these additional suggestions for maintaining and developing your P&T documents in mind:

- Institutions often require faculty to submit two CVs: a comprehensive vitae and one only including work for the tenurable year under review.

- Some universities require faculty to include narratives describing and discussing their research, teaching, and service. These narratives are typically two to three pages and are placed at the front of each section of the notebook. For example, the narrative related to scholarly research activities describes how the published manuscripts are consistent with a faculty's line of research. The narrative may also discuss each manuscript's contribution to the field of nursing and how other researchers in the field will use the information. In addition, the narrative may describe their specific contributions to manuscripts with multiple authors, impact factors, and the acceptance rates of the journals in which they published manuscripts.

- Narratives related to teaching often describe the quality of teaching and course evaluations. Within the narrative related to teaching, it is important discuss the following:

  a. The pedagogy underlying your instructional methods and techniques used.

  b. Any poor course evaluations and negative student comments. For example, if there is a consistent pattern to the type of negative student comments (e.g., students comment on a lack of feedback on an assignment across sections of the same course), it is important to address this within the narrative.

  c. How you use your course evaluations and student comments to enhance instructions. Demonstrate that you are responsive to student feedback.

  d. Any innovative instructional methods or assignments you implemented in your courses.

  e. Any teaching awards you have received.

  f. Indicate how your research and service activities inform and enhance your teaching.

- When writing an overview of your professional service, it is important to highlight your national service and how it affects the department, college, and university. For example, if you serve on an editorial board, describe how your service on the editorial board brings national recognition to the university. Take a similar approach when describing your service with national associations. Service on select department, college, and university committees also should be discussed. Choose a few high-profile committees (e.g., curriculum committee, Internal Review Board [IRB] committee, member of university senate, etc.), and discuss your contributions. Avoid listing every committee you have served on; the P&T committee will see them on your CV. Finally, indicate how your service enhances your research and teaching efforts.

- Narratives are very important, and you should spend a significant amount of time developing them. Most P&T committee members will read the narratives prior to reviewing your materials. Your narratives need to be clear, lack confusing terminology, and focus on helping P&T committee members outside the field of nursing understand the quality and impact of your contributions, especially in the areas of research and service. Once your P&T materials leave the department, faculty from other disciplines outside of nursing will likely be reviewing and making decisions based on your narratives and submitted materials.

Start new electronic folders for each academic year. That way, when you submit something or something is accepted, it immediately goes into that particular year's folders. Then, if you need to reference it for any reason, you know to go to that year's file.

Did you know that academic departments, colleges, and universities have to submit accreditation reports on a regular (e.g., biannual, annual) basis? You will frequently get requests for copies of your manuscripts, grants, student ratings/evaluations, student work samples, and so on to include in these reports.

The Curriculum Vitae

The CV is a document that highlights your life's work, education, work experience, scholarly accomplishments, continuing education, memberships, and so on. It is generally used in academia to reflect work and remains fluid as long as you are employed (Purdue Online Writing, 2016). We have not found any specific standards for the CV format. However, your institution more than likely has a format that everyone in the department/college/university is required to use. A great resource for compiling a CV is *The Curriculum Vitae Handbook*, by Anthony and Roe (1994).

Keep in mind these pointers related to CVs:

- Always be honest. Many P&T committees check the status of publications and presentations.

- Do not attempt to pad your CV. Members of the P&T committee will quickly recognize when you are attempting to do so. For example, do not include nonrefereed published manuscripts with refereed published manuscripts. Do not include nonprofessional service activities under professional service. Separate national and international presentations from state and regional presentations.

- It is also important to list all the courses you have taught. Do not omit a course because you received low student ratings. Most P&T committees will request that department chairs provide a copy of your course evaluations when they are reviewing your materials, even if you provide copies of your course evaluations in your notebook.

- Do not mix other publications (e.g., newspaper articles, newsletter articles, published abstracts, published conference proceedings, technical reports, etc.) with your refereed publications.

For an example of a curriculum vitae, see Appendix A.

Even among professional colleagues, there are different ways to approach keeping the CV up to date. This section discusses three different options. Note that we advocate for the last option (Option 3). Yet we know that faculty approach this differently, so we review several options. Regardless of when you update your CV, the process is the same.

> *Option 1: Yearly Updates*—At the end of the academic year, set aside several days to organize your work and then update your CV. This might be an option if you are not going to teach in the summer and you can focus on this process during your downtime. We caution you, though— other priorities can come up, and then you will be left printing documents and updating the CV very close to the due date.

> *Option 2: Semester Updates*—Throughout the semester, set aside an afternoon to update your CV. This might be a good option if you have carved out four to eight hours every four weeks during the semester. You can concentrate on getting items on a more regular basis than Option 1 allows. However, faculty who opt for this way to update their CVs often comment that other semester priorities come up, at which point updating the CV goes to the bottom of the priority list.

Option 3: Update Regularly—Update your CV immediately, when you have a new item to add. Take the few minutes to add it to your CV. This is the option that we recommend. Not only will your CV always be current; there is also a sense of accomplishment that comes with immediately adding your completed work to your CV.

The tenure documents and CV go hand in hand. When you turn in your materials to the P&T committee, you will be turning in one updated CV and all the supporting materials (e.g., tenure-line documents). Tenure-line documents are discussed in detail in the following section.

EXAMPLE PROCESS: SUBMITTING A MANUSCRIPT FOR POSSIBLE PUBLICATION

1. Save the submission verification in an electronic file and print a copy.

2. Save the submitted manuscript and the verification into your yearly tenure folder.

3. Immediately enter information into your personal CV and the institution's CV.

4. Upload any required documents (e.g., submission verification or submitted manuscript) into the digital CV or required digital reporting. The authors keep a printed copy of their manuscripts, IRB proposals, and grant proposals. Having a printed copy helps when developing "to do" lists, writing reports, providing updates to administration or to donors, etc.

5. Save the newly updated CV.

We recommend saving your CV in two places. Store one CV on your desktop and one in the cloud or on box. Sync them so that when one is updated, all saved copies are updated.

When saving your file, always include the date. You might be working with others, and all parties need to know which copy is the most recent.

A common mistake is not keeping the CV updated on a regular basis. Failure to update your CV with current information (e.g., manuscripts, memberships, and committees) will cause you to eliminate information and not give a full picture of your life's work. A simple tip for keeping your CV in "ready condition" is to take the time to add your work accomplishments as you complete them. This simple tip will help you keep your documentation organized and minimize last-minute attempts at trying to remember what you did months or even years ago. Adding the information as you complete it is a great habit to establish.

CURRICULUM VITAE (CV)

- ❏ Stay organized.
- ❏ Update with documents and accomplishments as you complete them.
- ❏ Review the CV regularly for errors or missing information.

Tenure-Line Documents

During your probationary period, all scholarly (publications, presentations, grants) work that you complete must be organized in a sequential manner for the P&T committee review. This may generally be accomplished by the tenure-line candidate's maintaining a notebook binder with dividers for each category being reviewed, such as teaching, teaching observations, scholarship (publishing, presenting your work at conferences, grants), service, your personal CV, and professional development. You might also be permitted to use an online reporting system (Danowitz, 2012).

Submitting your tenure-line documents via binders has two significant benefits. The first is that the documents neatly present your work. P&T committee members each receive a binder and can easily see each document without having to scan through an online reporting system. Secondly, you maintain the binder until it's ready for submission, so you have your printed work easily available for reference.

After your binders are reviewed by the department, college, and university P&T committees, they are typically returned to you. Binders can be costly, and some faculty tend to develop separate binders for each year of the seven-year probationary period. The cost of binders and of printing all your documents, manuscripts, grant proposals, and teaching evaluations can add up, and some institutions require faculty to reimburse the cost of printing. Find a safe place to store your binders so that they are protected from being lost, stolen, or damaged (fire or water damage).

Using Electronic Programs

Many universities are transitioning to paperless systems for tenure document submission. If you are using an electronic program, such as ePortfolio, the categories might be already created; in other systems, you might need to create specific categories that meet the requirements for your individual institution (Danowitz, 2012). Portfolios and ePortfolios are not just for reflection and progress tracking for students and educators but have also moved into other realms of the work environment (Danowitz, 2012; Lowenthal, White, & Cooley, 2011).

Whether you use notebook binders or digital reporting, they both have positive and negative aspects that you must consider. Regardless of the type of electronic program you use to help develop your portfolio, you must password-protect it.

In 2004, Hewitt believed tenure portfolios served three different purposes: a summative (demonstrating growth), reflective (review of personal experience) (Lin, 2008), and showcase device (marketing or promotional of accomplishments) (Lin, 2008) of the tenure-line candidate's progress over the probationary period. Your institution dictates the type and manner of the tenure documents that are developed and maintained.

Using electronic programs for your record-keeping might simplify the process, because then you are not copying a multitude of papers. However, you have to upload or scan your documents into the program. You should get into a habit of uploading your documents as you submit them, or at least on a weekly schedule. It is very easy for this process to become overwhelming if you don't do it on a regular basis. For instance, when you submit a manuscript to a peer-reviewed journal, you need to upload the abstract and a copy of the manuscript.

For grants, you need to include the assigned grant numbers from your institution's contracts and grants office. Generally, you should include all teaching evaluations, including comments from students, peers, and administration. Some electronic recording-keeping programs might be set up to automatically upload the evaluations and courses you've taught over the year. You will most likely have to manually upload all other documents. As a rule, this process should be quite simple, yet there may be some complications.

Some programs allow only one document to be uploaded per entry. For instance, you initially upload a copy of a submitted manuscript, but later the manuscript needs to be revised and re-uploaded, but the system allows only one copy of the manuscript to be uploaded in the individual entry. Furthermore, it's common knowledge that electronics fail at times, so you might experience a loss of your uploaded documents! You should do periodic checks to make sure all of your documentation is correct. In addition, there are some institutions that allow faculty to save documents on a flash drive or in the cloud.

As you can see, there's more than one option for tenure-line faculty to develop and save their documentation. Regardless of how you choose to maintain your documents, diligence in organization and time management is essential.

Chapter Checkup

❑ Do I understand why I need to keep my CV updated?

❑ Do I understand why I need to save and print my tenure-line documents?

❑ Do I know how my institution wants me to submit my yearly CV and documents (e.g., notebook binder or electronically)?

❑ Have I determined when I am going to update my CV (e.g., annually, each semester, or on a regular basis)?

❑ Do I understand what documents my institution requires (e.g., submission verifications, manuscripts, grant proposals, IRB proposals, etc.)?

❑ Have I developed my own steps and practices to keep myself organized?

References

Anthony, R., & Roe, G. (1994). *The Curriculum Vitae Handbook*. Iowa City, IA: Rudi Publishing.

Danowitz, E. S. (2012). On the right track: Using ePortfolios as tenure files. *International Journal of ePortfolio*. Retrieved from http://www.theijep.com/pdf/IJEP55.pdf

Hewitt, S. M. (2004). Electronic portfolios: Improving instructional practices. *Tech-Trends, 48*(5), 26–30.

Lin, Q. (2008). Preservice teachers' learning experiences of constructing e-portfolios online. *Internet and Higher Education, 11*(3/4), 194–200. doi:10.1016/j.iheduc.2008.07.002

Lowenthal, P., White, J. W., & Cooley, K. (2011). Remake/remodel: Using ePortfolios and a system of gates to improve student assessment and program evaluation. *International Journal of ePortfolios, 1*(1), 61–70.

Purdue Online Writing. (2016). Writing the curriculum vitae. Retrieved from https://owl.english.purdue.edu/owl/resource/641/1/

DOCTORAL DEGREES

ELEMENTS OF DOCTORAL DEGREES

1. PhD has a stronger focus on research and requires a dissertation.

2. EdD has a stronger focus on education and requires a dissertation.

3. DNP prepares the nurse for clinical practice with no dissertation requirement.

If you have not already earned a doctoral degree, it might be wise for you to consider the information presented in this chapter about the different doctoral degree types. The chapter focuses on discussing the different types of doctoral degrees and how they are accepted and function in higher education. Interestingly, nursing programs tend to hire an eclectic group of doctoral-trained individuals. Whereas some disciplines only hire individuals with a Doctor of Philosophy (PhD) degree, nursing programs tend to hire individuals with PhD, Doctor of Education (EdD), or Doctor of Nursing Practice (DNP) degrees.

Among these degrees, there are differences in educational preparation, dissertation or project focus, and faculty employment opportunities within universities and colleges. Consider these points regarding doctoral degrees:

- Although many doctoral programs offer similar core courses, some programs provide specialized coursework. For example, a program may be nationally recognized for training doctoral-level nurses with specialties in wound care. Prior to accepting a position at such an institution, be sure to confirm that you can pursue your own line of research if it is not consistent with the program's nationally recognized line of research.

- Faculty at an institution often determine the areas of specialization. For example, if two or three faculty at a school of nursing have been conducting research and publishing works on diabetes for more than 20 years, it is likely that doctoral students graduating from that program will also pursue similar lines of research once they graduate.

- The quality and types of research conducted by faculty at a school of nursing tend not to reflect the type of doctoral degree the faculty earn. Interestingly, whether faculty become excellent researchers and publish prodigiously seem more dependent on other variables (e.g., writing skills, knowledge of research design, knowledge of statistics, motivation, etc.) than on the type of doctoral degree they earned.

- Direct admits of students with baccalaureate degrees into a PhD nursing program is rare. Whereas other disciplines (e.g., psychology, education, biology, etc.) directly admit individuals with only a baccalaureate degree into their doctoral programs, doctoral programs in nursing often require some clinical experience and/or a master's degree.

Some universities will not hire faculty for tenure-track positions to work at the institution where they attained their doctorate, meaning that you might need to seek employment at another college/university. However, this written or unwritten policy may be more evident at major universities with a Carnegie Doctoral classification. The university may hire you into a full-time clinical or contract faculty position. The university may require you to work at another university for a period of time before it is willing to hire you into a tenure-track position. The philosophy is that graduates of their doctoral program need to establish themselves as researchers independent of the program from which they graduated. In addition, it is sometimes difficult to end a semester as a student and start the next semester as a colleague in that same department.

Nursing programs tend to hire faculty with a variety of degrees. This is likely due to the overall limited number of doctoral-level nursing training programs and the limited number of doctoral programs offering the PhD. Interestingly, many nurses will complete a master's degree in nursing and then pursue a doctoral degree in a closely related field (e.g., adult education, special education, mental health, health economics, etc.). The following sections discuss the different doctoral degrees in further detail.

Doctor of Philosophy (PhD)

Individuals completing a PhD typically complete three to four years of full-time coursework and research after earning their master's degree. With the PhD, there tends to be a stronger focus on taking research (e.g., research methods) and statistics courses with the goal of preparing students to not only consume the extant literature but also be able to contribute new knowledge by conducting rigorous research. PhD students are often expected to conduct research and publish, even prior to starting their doctoral dissertations. The dissertations can take several years to complete and are often expected to address a major issue within the profession.

The term *philosophy* means *love of wisdom* (Haidar, 2016). The PhD is considered a *terminal degree,* or the highest degree achieved, and it qualifies the person for a career in academia and/or research.

PhD candidates typically conduct original research, write the research results (the dissertation), complete written and comprehensive exams, and take oral exams to defend their research to a selected committee (Haidar, 2016).

Doctor of Education (EdD)

The EdD degree tends to focus on teaching, research, and determining solutions to address educational problems (Canipe, 2016). Most EdD programs are affiliated with colleges or schools of education. Compared to the PhD, students are not typically required to take as many research and statistics courses. However, it seems that the distinction between the PhD and EdD is becoming more difficult to discern. Depending on the selected program, earning an EdD prepares graduates to apply research and knowledge to organizations, leadership, and education problems and conduct original research (Teach.com, 2016).

Like the PhD programs, an EdD program may take three to six years of additional study beyond the undergraduate degree, and it culminates in a dissertation with the same requirements as the PhD with regard to conducting original research, completing written comprehensive exams, and orally defending the dissertation.

The Doctor of Nursing Practice (DNP)

The DNP is a terminal degree and is a relatively new practice doctorate in the area of professional nursing practice. As stated in Chapter 5, the intent of the DNP is to prepare nurse experts in population-based practice and to advance the education of nurses to the practice doctorate (American Association of Colleges of Nursing [AACN], 2004). There are lots of new DNP programs being developed in the United States, but there is also some confusion as to the intent of the DNP and where graduates may be employed.

 Grey (2013) points out that the intent of the DNP is to advance clinical practice, healthcare policy, and education. Grey also conveys that although the intent of the DNP-prepared nurse is to work in clinical practice, many nurses are now employed in nonrelated population-based settings.

How Your Degree Influences Promotion and Tenure

Unfortunately, other faculty outside of nursing often are confused regarding the credentials and different degrees associated with faculty within the school of nursing. Helping other faculty understand how the different degrees, training backgrounds, and research backgrounds influence the promotion and tenure expectations of faculty in schools of nursing is important. The following comments may be helpful for you to consider:

- Once you enter into a tenure-line position, whether you have a PhD, EdD, or DNP typically has no bearing on promotion and tenure decisions. Promotion and tenure decisions are based on how well you meet the teaching, research, and service expectations as outlined by your university.

- Universities are hiring individuals with DNP credentials into rigorous tenure-line positions. If the DNP program adequately prepared you to conduct research, you should be fine. However, if you completed only one or two research methods or statistics courses and/or did not complete a rigorous study (e.g., doctoral dissertation) while completing your degree, you likely will struggle to conduct research and publish.

- Many schools of nursing are so desperate for students that they will hire any faculty into tenure-line positions, even if they have minimal doctoral-level coursework in research methods and statistics. In fact, we have seen faculty hired into tenure-track positions without any refereed publications or national presentations. These faculty have to work very hard to establish a line of research and publish. It is not uncommon for these faculty to switch to full-time clinical or contract faculty positions within three to four years.

- Salary and merit raises are not typically linked to degree type. Here again, it is the faculty member's work that should determine salary and merit increases. However, if you are being offered a position and, during the negotiation, they indicate they cannot offer you as much due to your degree type, you might want to step back and reexamine the position.

- If your position is aligned with your degree type, make sure to clarify this during promotion and tenure decisions. For example, if you are a DNP, and you are in a tenure-line clinical faculty position, your requirements for promotion and tenure should be different compared to another faculty member in a tenure-line position that stresses research, teaching, and service. Make sure the different expectations are clearly indicated on your appointment letter, departmental promotion and tenure documents, and university promotion and tenure documents. When submitting your promotion and tenure materials, clearly outline the different requirements and how you meet them.

Chapter Checkup

❑ Do I understand the differences among the PhD, EdD, and DNP degrees?

❑ Do I understand how my degree will affect my tenure process?

❑ Do I understand that if my degree is a DNP, I might not be fully prepared for the rigor or requirements of research?

References

American Association of Colleges of Nursing (AACN). (2004). AACN position statement on the practice doctorate in nursing. Retrieved from http://www.aacn.nche.edu/publications/position/DNPpositionstatement.pdf. doi:10.3928/01484834-20101230-03

Canipe, S. (2016). How do I tell if I want an EdD or a PhD in education? *Walden University*. Retrieved from https://www.waldenu.edu/programs/education/resource/how-to-tell-if-i-want-an-edd-or-a-phd-in-education

Grey, M. (2013). The doctor of nursing practice: Defining the next steps. *Journal of Nursing Education, 52*(8), 462–465.

Haidar, H. (2016). What is a PhD? *TopUniversities.* Retrieved from http://www.topuniversities.com/blog/what-phd

Teach.com. (2016). EdD vs. PhD degrees. Retrieved from http://teach.com/how-to-become-a-teacher/get-educated/doctorate-in-education-edd/edd-vs-phd-degrees/

DEALING WITH POOR COURSE EVALUATIONS

ELEMENTS OF COURSE EVALUATIONS

1. Allows an opportunity for students to evaluate faculty

2. Offers an opportunity for faculty to use evaluations as constructive feedback

3. Allows the student to provide feedback on the course

4. Allows the faculty to review evaluations and improve teaching

Student evaluations, course ratings, and written comments are reviewed during the tenure process. When reviewing course evaluations, the department chair and promotion and tenure (P&T) committees often look for common themes (e.g., consistently low ratings on specific items, no clear course objectives, instructor availability, lack of feedback on assignments, etc.) that pop up during the probationary period. The department chair and department P&T committee also look to determine whether faculty are being responsive to student and faculty feedback related to their teaching.

Student Evaluations and the Tenure Process

There is no doubt that student course evaluations are an important consideration when faculty tenure documents are reviewed. And, as we have stated, more than likely you will be required to submit your student evaluations every year during the probationary process. However, there has been a debate surrounding the value that student evaluations bring to the faculty evaluation process.

Flaherty (2016) discusses that there is increasing evidence that student course evaluations are unreliable and may be biased, especially against female faculty. Sprague (2016) also points out that student evaluations show bias based on class expectations, race, gender, and age of the faculty and students.

> Student course evaluations are typically reviewed by the department chair and the college dean on a yearly basis, even with faculty who are promoted and tenured. Your students' course evaluations will likely be reviewed throughout your entire professional career.

Faculty believe that students also use evaluations to vent frustrations or to make personal comments about faculty (Patton, 2015). Stark (2013), at the University of California Berkeley, believes that student evaluations of faculty are basically popularity contests. In fact, Stark and Freishtat (2014) conclude in their study that although student evaluations have been used for years as a primary measure of teaching effectiveness—for promotion, tenure, and merit—the evaluations should be abandoned, because they actually do not measure teaching effectiveness. They conclude that comparing averages across courses, faculty, and departments does not make much sense.

Anecdotally, there has always been a long-standing discussion among faculty that student evaluations are influenced by grades (e.g., soft graders will earn higher rates), individual faculty perceptions, and class procedures. Some faculty believe there is a real disconnect in how evaluations are used for promotion and tenure and how generally useful they are (Patton, 2015).

Nevertheless, faculty should know how their institution views student evaluations and what weight, if any, is placed on student course evaluations. For example, if student course evaluations are more heavily weighted (e.g., 90%) compared to other forms of teaching evaluations (e.g., department chair course review, colleague course observation, and student outcomes), then a semester of poor student course evaluations could outweigh a positive teaching administrative evaluation, thereby resulting in a negative tenure decision for that year.

On a related side note, student ratings may be linked to your ability to earn yearly merit increases and promotion from associate to full professor. Many institutions place some sort of value on student course evaluations, and faculty must meet these minimum criteria to be considered for merit or promotion from associate to full professor. For example, on a five-point Likert scale, an institution may require that faculty receive student course evaluations that average 3.5 or better to be considered for merit. Likewise, to earn promotion from associate to full professor, the faculty must have student course evaluations that average 4.2 or better in the past two consecutive years.

Student course evaluations are generally completed online, anonymously, during the last two weeks of the semester. Some universities may still use paper versions, although these are becoming rare. Many evaluations are created with a Likert-type scale, giving students the opportunity to rate the overall course, including the content and faculty (e.g., instructor). In addition, students have an opportunity to write in comments. After the course has ended, faculty receive the results of the evaluations, including the written comments, but in most situations they are not allowed to respond to students.

EXAMPLE OF TYPES OF EVALUATION STATEMENTS

1. My instructor explains the course objectives clearly.

2. My instructor explains course content clearly.

3. My instructor provides timely feedback.

4. My instructor is available for questions or consultations (by phone, office hours, email, by appointment, or by videoconferencing).

5. The course has a clear grading system.

6. The course has clear objectives.

7. The course is effective at meeting the objectives.

Reviewing Student Evaluations

Reviewing student evaluations may be a little like going to the dentist to get that aching tooth dealt with—you know that you have to tend to it, but the treatment might be just as painful. You are not alone. Believe us when we say that we have all received a nasty comment from a student (and we know we are pretty awesome teachers!). No matter how good at teaching you are, there can always be room for improvement. Perfection is not a realistic goal—so let that go!

If you receive negative evaluations, your first reactions may be:

- *To be angry.* You may get angry and blame the students, even saying things (that you really do not mean) such as, "This group of students was just lazy. They didn't do anything" or "If it weren't for the students, I would really enjoy teaching" or "Students today aren't like when I was in school; they just don't respect the faculty. They are just rude."

- *To make excuses.* You might begin making excuses, and even lash out at others, to justify the poor evaluations. "I had a huge grant to get started this semester, so administration can't expect my evaluations to be good when they are over-working me" or "Well, this is a hybrid course. If I told my department chair once, I told her a thousand times—hybrid courses do not work" or "Those students could not learn their way out of a wet paper bag."

When you read your evaluations, keep an open mind, and put yourself in the students' position. As you read through the evaluations, look for common themes, especially themes across semesters (e.g., complaints about errors in the test key, no variety in assignments). Identify issues you can easily correct (e.g., missing items in syllabus, office hours not posted) versus issues that are large in scale (e.g., major curriculum issue). Weed out the items you do not own (e.g., bursar issue, other course issue), and disregard mean-spirited comments.

I have a leadership background (master's in business), so I view student evaluations very much like I did when I asked my direct reports to evaluate me. Meaning, I see my students very much as stakeholders. They absolutely should be able to evaluate me to offer constructive criticism. They pay my salary, after all! However, that does not give them the right to be hateful or abusive. Just because a student offers a suggestion or comment does not mean that I have to make a change. However, it is my responsibility to review the evaluations and follow up appropriately.
–Connie McIntosh

What if you receive really good evaluations? Look at them to decide whether there is anything glaring that still needs to be addressed in your class. For example, what if multiple students suggest that you offer a synchronized chat for your online students? This suggestion is a pretty low-hanging fruit that could easily be implemented. This suggestion alone may take your course from good to great.

Responding Constructively

We recommend that tenure-line faculty review their student course evaluations with their faculty mentor, at least for the first few semesters. Your mentor can help you interpret and process the reviews. Your mentor also can help identify student comments that you should address in future revisions of the course. If it's deemed appropriate, your faculty mentor will likely ask you a series of questions to help you better understand your teaching, course preparation, and grading processes. For example, are there any aspects of the comments that might be valid? Are there improvements that you can make to your instruction methods? Are you communicating effectively with students? You and your mentor could easily put together a disposition chart, like the one shown in Table 11.1.

TABLE 11.1.   TYPICAL DISPOSITION CHART

Nature of Comment	Recommended Action
Student complains about the way you dress.	No action needed; personal in nature.
Student says that your graphics are old and outdated.	Take a good look at your materials, and update them immediately.
Student claims to know where you live and will seek justice for unfair grade.	Report this to your department head and the university, no matter how unlikely you think the student is to follow up on the threat.

Nature of Comment	Recommended Action
Student claims that class is too difficult.	You are not required to make your class "easy" for students. But if there are consistent complaints of this nature, you should look at why these claims are made.
Student says you didn't offer office hours.	Verify that your office hours are listed on the syllabus.
Large numbers of students say that you are unapproachable.	Give careful consideration to this. If you deem this to be a possibility, correct this with action.
Student says that you are an awful teacher yet makes reference to another instructor's teaching style and references a different course.	Ignore, because it is unclear whether the student is really talking about you.
Student claims that you never respond to questions.	Give careful consideration to this. If it's true, put practices into place that make you available to students, and be sure to follow up with inquiries.

 If you receive threatening or dangerous comments, you need to report this to your department chair immediately. Your department chair will guide you through processes available at the college or university to address them. Always take these comments seriously, and report them immediately.

Receiving Consistently Poor Course Evaluations

If you consistently receive poor student course evaluations, your department chair will have to take steps to help you improve your teaching skills. Typically, the department chair and/or a senior faculty member will review your course syllabus, lectures, assignments, and exams and provide feedback. Someone might also conduct a classroom observation and provide feedback to you as well.

The department chair will likely recommend one or a combination of the following:

- Require you to attend workshops or training focused on enhancing your teaching.

- Develop and implement a remediation plan, which will include expected outcomes.

- Have you co-teach several courses with a seasoned instructor.

- Although this does not address the poor teaching results, he might reassign you to online courses only. However, we have seen department chairs pull faculty from teaching on-campus courses and reassign them to online courses without realizing that online courses are just as demanding as on-campus courses.

- Reassign you to clinicals to avoid on campus face-to-face courses. This is also not a great way to address and fix the issue.

- Request that you seek counseling. If the reasons for your poor evaluations are related to personal or family issues (e.g., currently going through a divorce) that are affecting your teaching abilities, the department chair may suggest counseling.

- Meet with someone to address time management.

It is important to listen to your department chair and to develop a plan together to improve your teaching skills. Although it can be embarrassing to receive poor student course evaluations, it is not uncommon to struggle during the first couple of semesters or even the first couple of years. Many doctoral programs do not provide instruction on how to be an effective teacher, and many doctoral programs do not even require students to teach while in the program. Therefore, many beginning faculty start academic positions without ever having taught a course. Some faculty are natural teachers, and some faculty have to work hard to be effective teachers.

TIPS FOR IMPROVING YOUR TEACHING

❏ Be energetic.

❏ Listen to what students are saying, and ask for input to improve the class.

❏ Be willing to adapt.

❏ Provide great stories that parallel your lecture material.

❏ Reflect on positive and negative aspects of the class dynamics.

❏ Offer diverse learning strategies/techniques for the variety of learners in the class.

❏ Engage the students with real-life situations.

❏ Be positive.

❏ Add some humor.

❏ Ask questions, and clarify often.

❏ Use technology to your advantage.

❏ Be a positive role model.

❏ Mix things up regularly.

❏ Expect participation.

❏ Ask good questions, and expect diverse answers.

Chapter Checkup

❏ Do I have a clear understanding of the student evaluation process?

❏ Do I understand how student evaluations are weighted in my tenure review?

❏ Do I know how to review my own student evaluations constructively?

❏ Do I understand how to review the student ratings and the student comments?

❏ Do I know how to prioritize any themes in my student evaluations?

References

Flaherty, C. (2016). Bias against female instructors. *Inside Higher Ed.* Retrieved from https://www.insidehighered.com/news/2016/01/11/new-analysis-offers-more-evidence-against-student-evaluations-teaching

Patton, S. (2015). Student evaluations: Feared, loathed, and not going anywhere. *Chronicle Vitae.* Retrieved from https://chroniclevitae.com/news/1011-student-evaluations-feared-loathed-and-not-going-anywhere

Sprague, J. (2016). The bias in student course evaluations. *Inside Higher Ed.* Retrieved from https://www.insidehighered.com/advice/2016/06/17/removing-bias-student-evaluations-faculty-members-essay

Stark, P. B. (2013). What exactly do student evaluations measure? *Berkeley Blog.* Retrieved from http://blogs.berkeley.edu/2013/10/21/what-exactly-do-student-evaluations-measure/

Stark, P. B., & Freishtat, R. (2014). An evaluation of course evaluations. *Science Open.* https://www.scienceopen.com/document/vid/42e6aae5-246b-4900-8015-dc99b-467b6e4?0

12

WORKING WITH YOUR MENTOR

ELEMENTS OF WORKING WITH YOUR MENTOR

1. Develops a trusted relationship between mentor and mentee

2. Ensures leadership from a senior faculty

3. Ensures guidance from senior faculty on the requirement of teaching

4. Ensures guidance from senior faculty on the requirement of scholarship

5. Ensures guidance from senior faculty on the requirement of service

This chapter addresses the importance of working with a faculty mentor. A *mentor* is in a leadership position and must be passionate about influencing others in the profession (Roussel, Thomas, & Harris, 2016). Mentors are very important to the overall success of a tenure-line candidate and should be chosen carefully to establish a healthy, trusting relationship.

The Mentor/Mentee Relationship

The mentor/mentee role is very important in building a relationship, developing leadership, improving communication, and nurturing professional attributes (American Organization of Nurse Executives [AONE], 2014). According to Roussel et al. (2016), mentoring is a relationship between a more experienced and competent role model (tenured faculty) and a less experienced (tenure-line) faculty where the tenured faculty serves as a counselor and resource person to help the tenure-line faculty develop professionally in teaching, scholarship, and service.

Selecting Your Mentor

The mentee (tenure-line) faculty must be a willing participant in the mentoring process; otherwise, the mentoring process will not work. Tenure-line faculty need to participate in goal planning and be willing to accept crucial feedback (Roussel et al., 2016). Because the tenure-line progression is usually a seven-year process, we cannot overstate how important it is to select your mentor carefully. The relationship needs to be well thought out prior to your entering a mentoring agreement. We are aware that in some departments, a mentor may be assigned and the mentee has no other option, but if you have the opportunity to select the mentor, be sure to give it careful consideration.

Consider these pointers when selecting your mentor:

- Avoid asking the department chair or another administrator to serve as a mentor. They are typically too busy, and it will be difficult for them to separate being your supervisor versus serving as your mentor.

- Select a mentor who has been at the university at least five years. If possible, select a mentor who recently attained promotion and tenure.

- Do not select someone you are related to or someone you are very close friends with to serve as your mentor. Although it is common for a mentor to become a very close friend, it is important at the start for the mentor to be able to provide you with unbiased advice.

Identifying Unofficial Mentors

Unofficial mentors are individuals who may not be in your own department, but who work with you throughout the tenure process in an unofficial capacity. You may want to seek out an unofficial mentor if your assigned mentor becomes uninterested (e.g., life circumstances change) or is too busy (e.g., travels) to work with you. When you look for an unofficial mentor, look for someone who:

- Has successfully completed tenure

- Is well respected at the university

- Is a seasoned educator

- Is an experienced researcher

The Role of the Mentor

The faculty mentor and tenure-line faculty mentee roles are different but should complement each other. Faculty mentors should be reviewing the tenure-line requirements for every year (year 1, year 2, and so on) of the probationary period and should hold you accountable to your individual goals.

When agreeing to be a mentor, that person is agreeing to put in the extra work, because mentorship is much more than just having coffee with an individual or identifying that a tenure-line faculty member has an issue. Rather, good mentoring is working with the individual for solutions to problems. In addition, your mentor should help you navigate through department, college, and university unwritten politics.

Additional Help From Mentors

Because you will be required to present your work at conferences, your mentor will help you determine the best conferences to which you should submit an abstract. Generally, abstracts are submitted for poster presentations and podium presentations. Some departments give equal credit to both styles of presentations, whereas others give more credit to podium presentations than to posters.

Your mentor should help you write the abstract and submit the work the first time but will probably expect you to be more independent for others. If you are not accustomed to presenting at conferences, your mentor might suggest that you be one of several faculty giving a podium presentation until you gain more confidence and experience. Don't be too hard on yourself after presentations, as it simply takes time and experience to gain confidence and develop a presentation style.

A good mentor serves as your counselor and resource person to help you develop professionally in teaching, scholarship, and service. Your mentor should be someone you can turn to with questions and for advice. If your institution doesn't require that you use an assigned mentor, choose your mentor wisely.

Chapter Checkup

❏ Do I have an understanding of what the mentor's role is?

❏ Do I have an understanding of what my role will be in the mentor-mentee relationship?

❏ Am I prepared to commit to what my mentor has asked me to do with regard to teaching, scholarship, and service?

❏ Do I understand that my mentor will be advising me, but I am the one who will be doing the work?

References

American Organization of Nurse Executives (AONE). (2014). Nurse executive competencies. Retrieved from http://www.aone.org/resources/leadership%20tools/nursecomp.shtml

Roussel, L., Thomas, P. L., & Harris, J. L. (2016). *Management and leadership for nurse administrators* (7th ed.). Burlington, MA: Jones and Bartlett Learning.

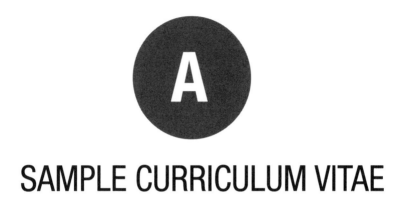

SAMPLE CURRICULUM VITAE

CURRICULUM VITAE
(01/11/2001)

Susan E. Jones

Jenkins State University
School of Nursing
Morgantown, NE 12345
Office: (123) 456-7890
sejones@morgantown.edu

BIOGRAPHICAL INFORMATION

Birth: Lint, NE - United States Citizen

Minority Status: Hispanic

EDUCATION

PhD Winter University
2001

> Nursing (Accredited)
> Specialty: Research Methodology
> Specialty: Community Nursing

> Doctoral Thesis Title: Cluster Analysis of the Nursing
> Satisfaction Scale With Nurses Working in Psychiatric Hospital

> Doctoral Mentor: Jane Smith, PhD

MA
1994

> Winter University

> Nursing

BA
1992

> Bass College at Bass Alaska

> Majors: Biology and Spanish

> Bass, Alaska

HONORS

Winter University Outstanding Faculty Service Award
1994

Instructor of the Year (School of Nursing)
1996

PROFESSIONAL AFFILIATIONS

American Nursing Association

PROFESSIONAL LICENSE

Registered Nurse, Nebraska (No. 1234)
Since 1993

PROFESSIONAL EXPERIENCE

08/1997–present   <u>Assistant Professor within the School of Nursing</u>,
University of South Lake, Brownville, Arkansas

08/1993–07/1997   <u>Registered Nurse at Sky Mountain Hospital</u>,
Whereabouts, Texas

PUBLICATIONS

Book

Jones, S. E. (1995). *A nurse's step-by-step guide to work satisfaction.* Indianapolis, IN: Sigma Theta Tau International.

Book Chapters

Jones, S. E. (in press). Working with psychiatric patients. In P. F. Loyd (Ed.), *A nurse's guide to working with psychiatric patients.* New York, NY: Smith.

Manuscripts Published in Refereed Journals—International/National

Jones, S. E., & Marcum, B. E. (1996). Medication administration: Following best practice. *Perspectives on Medication, 14*(1), 123–133.

Articles in Non-Refereed Journals

Jones, S. E. (1996, Summer). Cindy B. Clark: Interview with an icon. *The Nursing Specialist, 12*(7), 1 and 4.

Published Abstracts

List using proper citations abstracts and conference presentations that have been published in journals.

Reviews and Content Synopses

List using proper citations journal, article, instrument, and book reviews that have been published.

Technical Reports

List using proper format any technical reports written related to grants.

PRESENTATIONS

Symposiums Presented at National Professional Meetings

Jones, S. E., Wade, E. K., Smith, D. M., & Williams, R. S. (1995, April). *A collection of studies related to treating individuals with depression within the psychiatric setting.* Symposium presented at the annual meeting of the National Association of Mental Health Nurses, Washington, DC.

Presentations at National and International Professional Meetings

Jones, S. E. (1996, October). *Collaboration in curriculum development: A case study of a patient with depression.* Presented at the Annual Conference of the American Mental Health Nurse Association, Washington, D.C.

Papers Presented at Regional and State Meetings

List only presentations at regional and state meetings.

Invited Clinical Presentations

List all clinical presentations.

National, State, and Local Consultantships

1993 Consultant, Arkansas Division of Nursing Services

GRANTS/CONTRACTS

Grants/Contracts Awarded

1999–2000 (Total Amount=$200,000)

Arkansas State Federal Flow Through Granting Agency. Providing support services at the state level: Training nurses to work with depressed patients. October 1999–September 2000. Amount funded $86,152. (Principal Investigator.)

PROFESSIONAL SERVICE

Editorial and Reviewer Responsibilities

Editorial Board Member of *Journal of Attitudes in Nursing*, 2000–present
Ad Hoc Manuscript Reviewer for *Journal of Attitudes in Nursing*, 1998–2000

Service to Professional Organizations

National Association of Nurse Recruiting (National/International Organization)

Executive Board Member, 1999–2000

American Academy of Nurse Training

Past-President, 2000
President, 1999
President-Elect, 1998

Community Service

List all community (nonprofessional) service activities.

UNIVERSITY SERVICE

University

Curriculum Committee, 1999–2000
Library Subcommittee, 1997–1998

College

Curriculum Committee, 1999–2000
Travel Committee, 1997–1998
School of Nursing

Curriculum Committee, 1999–2000
Search Committee, 1997–1998
Applied Behavior Analysis and Autism Core, 2012–present
ABA and Autism Programs Director, 2011–2016

TEACHING

Graduate Courses Taught

Nursing 721: Psychiatric Nursing [Spring 2000]

Undergraduate Courses Taught

Nursing 321: Psychiatric Nursing [Fall 1997, Spring 1998, Fall 1998, Spring 1999]

Doctoral Dissertations

Student: John Smith
Topic: Pediatric Bipolar Disorder: Identification and Assessment of School Nurses
Service: Chair
Status: Completed July 1999

INDEX